Living a Caring-Based Program

Living a Caring-Based Program

Anne Boykin, Editor

National League for Nursing Press • New York
Pub. No. 14-2536

Printed in the United States of America

Contents

About the Authors   **vii**

Preface   **xiii**

Introduction   **xvii**

1. The Evolution of a Caring-Based Program   **1**
   Theris Touhy

2. Creating a Caring Environment for
   Nursing Education   **11**
   Anne Boykin

3. Nursing: A Discipline of Knowledge
   Grounded in Caring   **27**
   Marilyn E. Parker

4. The Shared Study of Nursing   **43**
   Diane Cope and Marilyn E. Parker

5. The Experience of Struggle, Freedom,
   and Growth   **65**
   Sherrilyn Coffman and Rozzano C. Locsin

6. The Experience of Being a Student in a
   Caring-Based Program   **79**
   Anita Beckerman, Anne Boykin, Susan Folden,
   and Jill Winland-Brown

Contents

7. Researching Experiences of Living Caring   **93**
Cheryl Tatano Beck

8. Prizing, Valuing, and Growing in a
   Caring-Based Program   **127**
Savina Schoenhofer and Sherrilyn Coffman

Appendix A: Past and Present Faculty
   Contributors   **167**

Appendix B: Courses in Curriculum   **169**

Appendix C: Undergraduate Program: Purpose
   and Objectives   **181**

Appendix D: Graduate Program: Purpose
   and Objectives   **185**

About the Authors

Anne Boykin is Dean, College of Nursing, Florida Atlantic University, Boca Raton, Florida. She received her master's degree in nursing from Emory University and her PhD in Higher Education and Administration from Vanderbilt University. She is President of the International Association for Human Caring, a former member of the NLN Board of Review, active in the American Association of Colleges of Nursing, a member of the Board of Directors of the Southern Council on Collegiate Education in Nursing, and numerous regional and state organizations. Dr. Boykin is an internationally known consultant for nursing education. She has published widely on caring in nursing including the 1993 co-authored NLN publication, *Nursing as Caring: A Model for Transforming Practice.*

Cheryl Tatano Beck is currently a Visiting Associate Professor at the University of Rhode Island College of Nursing. She received her master's degree in maternal-newborn nursing from Yale University. She is also a certified nurse-midwife. Cheryl went on to receive her Doctor of Nursing Science degree from Boston University. For the past 15 years, she has been teaching on the baccalaureate, master's, and doctoral levels of various universities such as Florida Atlantic University and the University of Michigan. Cheryl is actively involved in both quantitative and qualitative research. Her research endeavors have included women's temporal experiences during the childbearing cycle, caring within a nursing program, and postpartum depression. She has authored over 40 articles. In November 1993, she was inducted into Fellowship in the American Academy of Nursing.

Anita Beckerman, Assistant Professor of Nursing, Florida Atlantic University, began her basic nursing education in a generic master's Program, receiving her master of science degree from Pace University and New York Medical College in 1979. Upon graduation, she was an Adult Nurse Practitioner in a primary clinic of a municipal hospital. At the same time, she continued her graduate studies at Teacher's College, Columbia University, receiving her Ed.D. in 1983. She is certified by the American Nurses' Association as both a Gerontological and Adult Nurse Practitioner. Her research and publication interests are in the area of gerontology and adult health. She was the recipient of a research grant award from the Florida Nurses' Foundation in 1992 for her study on hope in the elderly. Currently, Dr. Beckerman also holds a position as Adjunct Nurse Researcher at the Miami Veteran's Affairs Medical Center.

Sherrilyn Coffman is Associate Professor, College of Nursing, Florida Atlantic University. A graduate of Indiana University, Dr. Coffman's major area of interest is nursing care of children and families. She teaches undergraduate students in pediatric and obstetric clinical areas, and graduate students in the area of family nursing. In 1992, she received the Award for Excellence in Undergraduate Teaching from the College of Nursing at Florida Atlantic University. Her area of nursing practice is neonatal intensive care and pediatrics. With a research focus on families, she has studied new parents' relationships and social support, families and natural disasters, and needs of families with chronically ill children. She was named the 1992 3M Health Care Scholar by the American Nurses Foundation for her study, "Nurse and Family Experiences in Home Care." Active in Sigma Theta Tau International, she has served as Iota Xi Chapter President, Region 7 Leadership Extern, and member of the International Library Scientific Committee.

Diane Cope obtained her PhD in Nursing from the University of Miami and is a Visiting Assistant Professor in the College of Nursing at Florida Atlantic University. Diane's commitment to the caring philosophy originated from advanced study of the Humanistic Theory proposed by Paterson and Zderad (1978) and from her interests in women's health and oncology nursing. She has worked extensively with women experiencing breast cancer. This involvement has been the impetus for research focusing on breast cancer screening behaviors, breast cancer support groups, and the experience of breast cancer survivorship. Diane's present research, involving family members of breast cancer survivors, is aimed at gaining a greater understanding of this experience to foster caring for women with breast cancer.

Susan L. Folden was an Assistant Professor at Florida Atlantic University from 1986 to 1993. She received her bachelor's and master's degrees from the University of Akron and her PhD in Nursing from the University of Miami. Her research and publications are focused on persons experiencing chronic illness. She is also the Sigma Theta Tau Region 7 Communications Coordinator.

Rozzano C. Locsin obtained his PhD in Nursing from the University of the Philippines College of Nursing in 1988. He is a certified gerontological nurse. His research and publications topics include: effects of music on postoperative pain, caring and curing orientations of nurses and physicians, time experiences among adult and elderly clients, and, currently, technological competence as expression of caring in nursing. His contemporary presentation of "illustrating music as aesthetic expression of caring in nursing" forged his interests in nursing, music, and pain. He recently completed a two-month consultancy project in the Philippines focusing on nursing curriculum and the development of conceptual/organizational frameworks in nursing. This was through the auspices of the United National Development Program (UNDP), specifically, the Transfer of Knowledge through Expatriate Nationals (TOKTEN) program.

Marilyn E. Parker, Associate Professor of Nursing, received her master's degree from Catholic University of America and her PhD from Kansas State University. She has worked for many years, in varied settings, with nurses in development and use of nursing theory in nursing education, practice, and administration. She is editor of *Nursing Theories in Practice* (1990), and *Patterns of Nursing Theories in Practice* (1993), both published by the National League for Nursing, and is co-founder and editor of *Nightingale Songs,* a forum for nurses to share reflections on their nursing. Her research program is focused on the study of nursing values and nursing practice and administration strategies. Innovative nursing philosophies and methods of inquiry are outcomes of the research. She is also a potter and has participated with nurses in developing ways of aesthetic knowing in nursing using clay and other media for recreating nursing situations.

Savina Schoenhofer is an Associate Professor in the Florida Atlantic University College of Nursing. Her master's degree is from Wichita State University and her PhD is from Kansas State University. She is co-founder of *Nightingale Songs,* a publication of nurses' creative writings. Dr. Schoenhofer established the Nursing Research Development Network, a collaboration of nurses in practice and education settings which has created an agenda for regional nursing research. Her publications have been in the areas of nursing home management, nursing values, caring, and touch as a medium for nursing in critical care settings. She is co-author of the 1993 NLN publication, *Nursing as Caring: A Model for Transforming Practice.*

Theris Touhy, Visiting Assistant Professor, College of Nursing, Florida Atlantic University, received her master's degree in nursing care of the aged from Northern Illinois University in 1979. She had the privilege of being on the original nursing faculty at the inception of the program of study in nursing at Florida Atlantic University in 1980. In both full- and part-time roles, she has maintained, over the past 13 years, an ongoing commitment to the development of a caring-based program. She is a Clinical Specialist in Gerontological Nursing and has many years of experience as an educator and nurse administrator at Manor Pines Convalescent Center in Fort Lauderdale. Areas of interest and research include strategies to enhance caring behaviors of students of nursing and practicing nurses toward the aged; the concept of nursing home as home for nursing; reminiscence group work with the institutionalized aged; and nursing with the memory-impaired person.

Jill Winland-Brown is an Associate Professor in the Florida Atlantic University College of Nursing. She received her master's degree from Boston College and her Ed.D. from Florida

Atlantic University. She worked for 10 years in critical care, staff development, and in supervisory positions. She attended a postdoctoral Intensive Bioethics Course at the Kennedy Institute of Ethics at Georgetown University. Areas of research and publication cover the lifespan and include ethics, caring in the practice settings, disabled nurses and camp nursing.

Preface

This timely publication offers a description of community building within the College of Nursing at Florida Atlantic University. Nursing education programs have a reputation of being demanding, difficult, and exhausting. Since the education process is the way students are socialized into the culture of nursing, it is the obligation of faculty to create an environment in which students come to know each other as colleagues who are free to express their uniqueness. This book describes the evolution and living of a caring-based program grounded in foundational beliefs and values of person and centered in caring.

Although this program resides in a tradition structure, governance moves away from hierarchial approaches and centers on principles supporting emancipation and transformation leadership. Ways of being with each other acknowledge and value the contributions of all individuals. A caring atmosphere encourages dialogue, debate, and different ways of knowing for faculty and students.

The curriculum is based on the discipline of nursing grounded in caring. It is viewed as the shared study of nursing. Students and faculty bring to class nursing situations that are relived and studied. In this way, content of the discipline is discovered and discussed. This approach appropriately employs content from other disciplines, such as the medical sciences, as empirical knowledge to understand nursing situations but not as the content of the discipline of nursing.

Faculty diversity, polemics, and dynamics are recognized and dealt with as part of the struggle, support, and growth inherent in caring. Faculty-faculty relationships require balancing the need for expression, maintaining integrity, being part of a whole, recognizing and valuing differences, and being willing to debate and dialogue while being supported, connected, and understood. Faculty evaluation guidelines are viewed as continuously unfolding, but most important is how faculty are with each other in the evaluation process. The context of scarce resources, competition to further careers, and the tenure versus nontenure issues make a commitment to caring as a moral obligation a very real challenge. Salary awards and tenure are not guaranteed but are determined through dialogue attempting to relate understandings of quality, suitability, and contributions. Evaluation is viewed as prizing, valuing, and growing.

The successful indictor or outcome for a caring-based program is the students' lived experiences. These experiences validate the efforts of faculty as students come to know self as a caring person. Coming to know self as a caring person is reflected in the study of nursing situations as they learn to respond, think critically, value self and others, and make nursing practice decisions/judgements based on caring.

The writings in this book demonstrate the importance of the environmental context and the need to pay attention to the whole in order to create a climate for learning, productivity, and scholarship. Caring can serve as a basis for nursing education, research, and practice; caring creates a space where people can contribute, grow, and be rewarded.

The challenge of creating a caring community for faculty and students is ever present. The nursing faculty at

Florida Atlantic University has accepted and is meeting this challenge. The writing of this book provides the opportunity to share with colleagues their knowledge, experiences, and ways of knowing and being in a caring-based program.

Joyce P. Murray, EdD, RN, CS
Associate Dean for Academic Affairs
Graduate Program Coordinator and Professor

Introduction

The stimuli for this book were the many questions raised by colleagues as to the nature of a caring-based program. The focal question was what does it mean to center a program of study in caring? This book attempts to illustrate the living of a caring-based program in nursing education.

We, like many nursing faculties, have struggled over the last decade to discover ways of teaching and learning nursing that truly reflect content and processes of the discipline. It became clear to the faculty that we must risk new ways of teaching nursing if our values and beliefs of nursing were to be lived out.

One of our faculty's major assumptions is that all persons are caring by virtue of their humanness. Understanding this assumption is essential to understanding our program of nursing education. This assumption does not intend to imply that all acts are caring, but it does intend that the potential for caring exists in each person in each moment—caring is a quality of being human. Understanding the generic sense of caring is essential to creating caring environments. This understanding guides all relationships as we come to know self and other as caring person. Therefore, the generic understanding of caring is an important link to understanding caring as uniquely lived in nursing.

Chapter 1 of this book offers a perspective on the unfolding of this program of nursing grounded in caring. Major factors influencing our understanding of caring are identified and processes used to uncover the essence of the discipline are described.

In Chapter 2, the beliefs and values which foster the creation of a caring environment for nursing education are presented. Examples are provided of how commitment to caring grounds all decisions and interactions inherent in the role of dean. A new organizational structure (circular not hierarchical in design) is introduced as a design which celebrates cherished values.

Chapter 3 describes the faculty's view of nursing as a discipline of knowledge and professional practice. Conceptions of person and nursing which ground nursing thought and inquiry are shared. The idea of nursing situation is presented as a way to study, develop, and organize content of the discipline.

Chapter 4 focuses on the shared study of nursing, more traditionally called the curriculum. Nursing situations are discussed and numerous examples add clarity to understanding this approach to teaching and learning nursing. The use of Carper's patterns of knowing to enhance the study of nursing situations are described.

Chapter 5 reveals the experience of being a faculty or staff member in a caring-based program. Struggles are balanced by satisfactions which include experiencing connectedness, support and respect, as well as personal freedom, sense of wholeness and growth.

Chapter 6 focuses on the experience of being a student in a caring-based program. Stories (from generic and registered nurse undergraduate students as well as graduate students) describe how they came to know themselves as caring persons and the meaning of this to their practice of nursing.

Introduction

Chapter 7 presents three phenomenological studies which investigated the meaning of caring in this program. The studies focused on student-faculty caring, student-student caring, and faculty-faculty caring experiences.

Chapter 8 approaches evaluation as the prizing, valuing and growing in a caring-based program. Central to evaluation is the assumption that the nature of being human is to be caring and persons are free for choosing values, aspirations and desires which give meaning to living. All aspects of the program are addressed and many examples reflecting caring values are provided.

I remain grateful to all persons who courageously risked freeing themselves in order to envision and experiment with another paradigm for nursing education. Each faculty person who in his or her own special way stroked their artist's brush across the creation of this program is acknowledged in Appendix A. We humbly offer to you our experiences of creating and living a caring-based program with the hope that it will stimulate thought regarding the nature of teaching and learning the discipline of nursing.

Anne Boykin

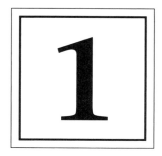

The Evolution of a Caring-Based Program

Theris Touhy

LIFE'S RAINBOW
Sheila Banani

Beginnings are lacquer red
　　fired hard in the kiln
　　of hot hope

Middles, copper yellow
　　in sunshine,
　　sometimes oxidize green
　　with tears, but

Endings are always indigo
　　before we step
　　on the other shore.*

* From: *When I am an old woman I shall wear purple,* edited by Sandra Martz, Papier Mache Press, Watsonville, California, 1987.

*I*n this chapter, I offer a particular perspective on the evolution of the nursing program at Florida Atlantic University. Having had the personal and professional good fortune of being a member of the nursing faculty at the inception of the program, and of maintaining an ongoing role in teaching and program development over the past 13 years, I am privileged to discuss the foundations of our current beliefs about nursing. In this regard, Mayeroff's (1971) recognition—that to care for another person, ideal, or idea is to help the other grow—is important. At Florida Atlantic, we were entrusted with caring for an idea of nursing. It was with great passion for nursing that we began the process of caring for that idea and helping it to grow.

In the late 1970s, the South Florida community served by Florida Atlantic University was growing rapidly. Because hospitals were seeking nurses with baccalaureate preparation in the discipline, practicing nurses in the community wanted to further their education and obtain baccalaureate and higher degrees in nursing. No public university in the area at that time offered a program of study leading to the bachelor's degree in nursing. Nonetheless, with the community advocating a need for nurses prepared at the baccalaureate level, in 1977 a program proposal was approved by the Florida Board of Regents. While no state funding was made available to initiate the program, community commitment to baccalaureate nurse preparation was so strong that several local donors provided start-up money. Under the leadership of Dr. Robert Huckshorn (Dean of the College of Social Science) and with guidance and consultation from nursing leaders in the community hospitals, from the junior college nursing programs in the area, and from the deans of baccalaureate programs within the state, program development began. In 1979, Florida Atlantic University, at that time an upper-division university within the state university system, began the upper-division nursing program for registered nurses under the auspices of the College of Social Science. A Consultant Director and four newly prepared master's degree nurses were appointed as faculty to teach the ten very competent and courageous registered nurses who enrolled in the fledgling nursing program.

We were blessed with an opportunity that allowed us freedom to create our concept of nursing and to explore innovative teaching strategies. We were supported and encouraged to dialogue on and study nursing. We were not yet aware of the many implications of our task, nor were we bound by what had come before. Our talented students were leaders in the nursing community and masters of their skill, and they had achieved a high level of success in the profession. They challenged us to articulate what they needed to learn about nursing. They forced us to continually think about nursing as a *concept*, apart from skills, techniques, and the medical model in which we had all been schooled. This was the task we faced as we began to study nursing and the knowledge needed by today's nurse. We shared our ideas on what was important in nursing practice and our hopes and dreams for how nursing practice could be improved. As we studied nursing, we began to filter nursing from non-nursing in an effort to articulate what it was in nursing that made a difference in the lives of people.

Among our early influences were the values and teaching work of Sid Simon and Jay Clark (1975) and Diane Ustal's (1977) work on values clarification in nursing. As a result, one of the earliest courses developed was Values Clarification, in which both student and faculty were given the opportunity to reflect and dialogue on values and valuing in nursing. Our teaching–learning philosophy was one of openness and mutuality, which yielded a healthy respect for learning from each other. We learned and taught the theory of Martha Rogers (1970) and the applications of the theory by her student,

Delores Kreiger (1981). The concepts of holistic nursing were explored, and the importance of nursing self and other for health was embraced. Discovering the works of Leininger (1981), Watson (1979), and Zderad and Patterson (1989) was like opening the best present under the Christmas tree. Caring for self and other emerged as an essential framework for nursing. With the addition of more experienced scholars and educators to the faculty, the dialogue on caring as a concept of great depth in the discipline took on new dimensions. We realized that there was much to know, and we were excited by the possibilities.

In 1982, the generic program began; in 1984, initial accreditation by the National League for Nursing was sought. Our curriculum, like many others at that time, was organized using a general systems theory framework. Through a self-study process, the faculty began to identify those aspects of the philosophy and, particularly, the framework that did not fully express where we were in our thinking about nursing. With accreditation knocking at the door, our collective wisdom told us to postpone undertaking major curriculum changes. (I wonder how many people who read this book will find this to "ring true" with them.) October 1984 came, the site-visitors left, and initial accreditation of the baccalaureate program was granted in December 1984. At approximately this same time, the nursing program received a major gift (which the state matched) from an individual donor to create the million-dollar Christine E. Lynn Eminent Scholar Chair. The purpose of this Chair was to advance knowledge in the discipline.

This was an exciting time. Faculty began to ask difficult questions, such as: Do we want to continue teaching nursing as we have been, or shall we take the risk and ask the question—what is the content of the discipline that should be taught? All faculty knew that the classroom content being taught was predominantly medical science and that some content of the discipline wasn't being addressed. We struggled to come to know what, in fact, *is* the content of the discipline.

The process of discovery began by evaluating the outlines for the current classes. The first step was easy: all the content considered not nursing-specific was sorted out. A decision was made to place all of the pathophysiology and pharmacology content into a pair of 4-credit courses. What content should fill these huge holes? What belonged in the content of the discipline?

We began to meet regularly and, by sharing our individual stories of nursing practice, we began to believe that if they were shared with students the content of nursing would be known. (This process was long, confusing, exciting, scary, and continuous. Omission of its details should not portray the process as simple and without painful struggles.) The decision was made to experiment with teaching the content of nursing through the use of nursing situations (defined as the lived experiences in which the caring between nurse and client fosters well-being). (Nursing situations and the process of teaching are described in Chapter 4.)

Throughout our dialogue, the importance of caring as a unique concept in nursing continued to unfold. Many factors nurtured and influenced the growth of this concept. Mayeroff's book, *On Caring* (1971), has been and continues to be a required text in our program because it offers a generic way of knowing self and other as caring person. Mayerhoff's major ingredients of caring were in place: knowing, alternating rhythms, trust, hope, courage, humility, patience, honesty. We were given the freedom and support to study nursing. We had the gift of time to reflect, to dialogue, to read and research. We had bright and committed students eager to learn. We were free to experiment—and make mistakes. We were humble enough to know that we had much to learn. We nurtured and supported each other, and we developed into a caring community of nurses. We cared for our idea of nursing, and we welcomed with joy new members who would assist us in our exciting work.

> This then is the basic pattern of caring, understood as helping the other grow; I experience the other as an extension of myself and also as independent and with the need to grow; I experience the other's development as bound up with my own sense of well-being; and I feel needed by it for that growing. I respond affirmatively and with devotion to the other's need, guided by the direction of its growth. I commit myself to the other and to a largely unforeseeable future. In caring for the other, I actualize myself. (Mayeroff, 1971, p. 9)

Patterson and Zderad's book, *Humanistic Nursing* (1988), has also had a significant influence on the evolution of the curriculum. Their work exquisitely addressed the phenomenon of nursing; their ideas of nursing situations and call and response seemed to fit with our concept of nursing. Although individual faculty were at various points in their understanding of caring as unique in nursing, there was a common commitment to the development of this idea. The works of many other scholars were brought forward for ongoing dialogue. Our faculty did not ascribe to any particular work; instead, they created their own statements of belief on caring. The patchwork pieces of caring in nursing were cut, placed, and stitched together in different ways, rearranged again and again, until they started to become a beautiful whole quilt.

Following are excerpts from the original philosophy (1984) as well as the current philosophy. They indicate the movement of our thinking related to caring over the past ten years:

The goal of professional caring is to assist the individual, family, group, community, and society in attaining their maximal potential for health. (1981)

The foundation for professional caring is the blending of humanistic, scientific, and nursing theories. Humanistic caring is the creative, intuitive, and cognitive aspects of the helping process. (1981)

The goal of nursing is the promotion of the process of being and becoming through caring. (current)

Caring is not unique to nursing, but is unique in nursing. Caring in nursing is a mutual human process in which the nurse artistically responds with authentic presence to a call from a client. (current)

The integralness of caring to the practice of nursing has become more explicit. The focus of nursing today is centered on coming to know persons in the moment and on nurturing their being and becoming through caring. The philosophy of our program reflects the work of nursing's artists.

Our program's philosophy is given here in its entirety, lest there be misinterpretations:

The faculty of the College of Nursing believes the values and goals of higher learning and supports the Florida Atlantic University mission of education, scholarship, and service. Fundamental beliefs concerning Person, Nursing, and Learning Environment express the values and guide the endeavors of the faculty.

PERSON. The person is a uniquely human individual connected in oneness with others and the environment in a caring relationship. The nature of being human is to be caring. To be human is to be free for choosing values, aspirations, and desires which give meaning to living and reflect well-being. Well-being is creating and living the meaning of life. The well-being and becoming of persons, families, groups, communities, and societies are fostered through caring relationships and interrelationships with the environment.

NURSING. Nursing is a discipline of knowledge and a field of professional practice. The goal of nursing is the promotion of the process of being and becoming through caring. Caring is not unique to nursing, but is unique in nursing. Caring in nursing is a mutual human process in which the nurse artistically responds with authentic presence to a call from the client. The experience of nursing takes place in nursing situations: lived experiences in which the caring between nurse and client fosters well-being. Valid scholarship and practice in nursing require creative integration of knowing and caring. Nursing makes a unique contribution because of its special focus. Nurses participate with other disciplines and professions in the advancement of human understanding and betterment in personal and communal living within a global environment.

LEARNING ENVIRONMENT. Beliefs about learning and environments which foster learning are derived from an understanding of person, the nature of nursing and nursing knowledge, and the mission of the University. Learning involves the creation of understanding in the integrated appreciation of knowing within a context of value and meaning. A supportive environment for learning is a caring environment. A caring environment is one in which all aspects of the human person are respected, nurtured, and celebrated.

GRADUATE EDUCATION. The Faculty of the College of Nursing believes that graduate education in nursing must provide content which is explicit nursing knowledge and which is advanced in depth and scope beyond the beginning general focus of an undergraduate program. Students of advanced nursing are recognized as increasingly self-directed scholars with specific learning needs to support independent, collaborative nursing practice based on detailed, complex nursing knowledge. The learning environment for graduate study emphasizes collegial relationships with faculty and graduate students from nursing and other disciplines. Advanced scholarship in nursing takes place within the context of Nursing as a discipline and profession.

Before concluding this chapter, I would like to update our history to the present. Today, we are a College of Nursing with 19 full-time faculty, several part-time faculty, an Eminent Scholar, 200 upper-division undergraduate students, 200+ prerequisite students, over 100 graduate students, and 4 full-time staff. The graduate program began in Fall 1988 and received initial accreditation in 1991. In 1990, the Division of Nursing within the College of Social Science received the necessary support to become a free-standing School of Nursing. During the Spring 1991 legislative session, the President of the University, Dr. Anthony Catanese, processed to the Board of Regents paperwork necessary for us to become a College of Nursing. Our hope is that we will soon be approved to offer a PhD in Nursing and open a Center for Research and Caring in Nursing.

The work described here has been done with love and devotion. It is not completed, and the continuing creation of the whole out of pieces continues to be exciting and challenging. The concept of caring and the development of nursing knowledge related to caring in nursing continue to develop. We remain committed to caring for our idea and helping it to grow. We share our work in the hope that it will in some way be meaningful to our readers' own efforts.

REFERENCES

Kreiger, D. (1981). *Foundations for holistic health nursing practices: The renaissance nurse.* Philadelphia: J. B. Lippincott Co.

Leininger, M. (1981). *Caring: An essential human need.* Thorofare, NJ: Slack.

Mayeroff, M. (1971). *On caring.* New York: Harper & Row.

Patterson, J., & Zderad, L. (1988). *Humanistic nursing.* New York: National League for Nursing.

Rogers, M. E. (1970). *An introduction to the theoretical basis of nursing.* Philadelphia: Davis.

Simon, S. B., & Clark, J. (1975). *More values clarification: Strategies for the classroom.* San Diego: Pennant Press.

Ustal, D. (1977). Searching for Values, *Image, 9*(1), pp. 15–17.

Watson, J. (1979). *Nursing: The philosophy and science of care.* Boston: Little, Brown.

Creating a Caring Environment for Nursing Education

Anne Boykin

*T*his chapter presents the beliefs and values that ground the living of a caring-based program for nursing education. The words "caring-based program" are carefully chosen. It is the author's belief that it is not possible to live a caring-based curriculum if the foundation for the program is anything other than caring. Although the curriculum focuses on caring as uniquely expressed in nursing, caring in a broad sense guides a way of being.

I had been a faculty member for two years prior to assuming administrative responsibilities for this program. The program was small, and no faculty were tenured. Among us, the love of nursing was a common bond. It was an ideal situation for "nursing" a dream, and my dream was to create:

- A context for the study of nursing in which the beauty and special gifts of each person would be known and valued;
- An environment in which discourse on the nature of the discipline would occur openly, freely, and respectfully;
- A program of study grounded in the discipline and practice of nursing.

The philosophy of this program has been stated in Chapter 1. The beliefs about *person* expressed in the philosophy should guide the way of being with self and others. These are some of the basic philosophical tenets about person that directly guide our way of being and influence the living of a caring-based program:

- The nature of being human is to be caring.
- To be human is to be free for choosing values, aspirations, and desires which give meaning to living and reflect well-being.
- Well-being is creating and living the meaning of life.

*   *   *

- A caring environment is one in which all aspects of the human person are respected, nurtured, and celebrated.

"The nature of being human is to be caring" is indeed a powerful tenet because it declares that all persons are caring. There was much dialogue among faculty prior to the inclusion of this belief in the philosophy statement. The struggles included the obvious questions: How can it be said that all persons are caring when acts of some persons in society are often so contradictory to this description? Are persons innately caring? Can caring be taught? What does it mean to be caring? Roach's (1984) description of the entailments of caring was helpful in deepening the faculty's understanding of the human quality of caring. Roach stated that caring entails the capacity to care; it calls forth this ability in ourselves and others, and the response to something or someone that matters actualizes the ability to care. Given this basis, we are, by nature of being human, caring; however, not every act of a person reflects the calling forth of this ability.

Commitment to this expressed belief requires a particular way of being with self and other. A commitment to caring directs all actions; it obligates us to know self and other as caring person. Mayeroff's caring ingredients (1971, pp. 13–28), which have provided another framework for both faculty and students to use in order to know self as caring person, are described below:

- Knowing—knowing explicitly and implicitly; knowing that and knowing how, knowing directly and knowing indirectly.

- Alternating rhythms—having the ability to move from wider to narrower perspectives and to develop an honest understanding of other.

- Patience—not waiting passively for something to happen; instead, participating with the other and giving fully of ourselves; enlarging our living space—the space in which we think and feel.

- Honesty—trying to see truly.

- Trust—allowing the other to grow in his or her own special way.

- Humility—being willing to learn more about self and others.
- Hope—endorsing the present as being alive with possibilities.
- Courage—being ready to go into the unknown, to take risks, to make decisions with a commitment to caring.

Faculty and students strive together to know self and other as caring person. Questions consistently asked are:

- Who am I as caring person?
- How is caring being expressed in the moment?

Mayeroff's caring ingredients served as a stimulus to heighten the understanding of self and other. Other questions emerging from the use of this framework include:

- Who am I as student of professional nursing?
- What are my hopes and dreams?
- How do I express my uniqueness and caring moment-to-moment?
- How do I express my uniqueness in the role of faculty? of student?
- How can I free myself to become what I truly can become?
- How do I support others as they live caring in their unique way?
- How do I see myself? Do others see me in the same way?
- Am I open to honestly knowing self and other?

- If the response of other is honest, is this a reflection of caring?
- How do my actions demonstrate my respect for other? my willingness to allow other to grow in his or her own time and way?
- How do my actions reflect my trust that other will grow in his or her own time and way?
- How is humility expressed?
- How do my actions reflect hope in the moment?
- Am I willing to take necessary risks? to use my imagination?

Because the development of caring is a process of life, both students and faculty are in a continual search to better know self. The importance of knowing self as caring and of caring for self cannot be overemphasized. This knowledge changes how we are in our day-to-day living. It influences and changes our way of relating. Establishing relationships rooted in a commitment to caring necessitates coming to know other as person expressing caring in the moment. This commitment carries with it a desire to know other as colleague; to support the sharing of knowledge, values, and beliefs; to understand other's views; to search for new solutions to problems from a caring perspective; to share responsibilities and authority; and to always treat each other in a manner reflective of the specialness of person.

The process for knowing self as caring is ongoing, and strategies to accomplish this knowledge vary. Faculty participate in retreats focused on knowing self as caring person. In open dialogue, we share stories of how we know self and other as caring. Openly discussed also are our hopes and dreams of growing through caring. For the entire time students are enrolled in the professional phase of the program, they focus on coming to better know themselves as caring, unique persons. Because the development of caring is a process of life, both students and faculty are in a continual search to know self better. It is the faculty's belief that, because the practice of nursing is mutual and interactional (involving both the client and nurse), it is incumbent on us in the teaching of nursing to focus deliberately on helping students know who they are and to support them as they seek to grow in their own unique ways.

In many nursing programs and in bureaucracies in general, however, the organizational structure is not one in which these beliefs are freely expressed. Organizational structures reflect bureaucratic values and explicitly portray a way of being with and relating to people. The existing concept of hierarchy implies a top, a bottom, competition, levels, and positions of power. From this perspective, it is difficult for each member in an organization to risk being authentic, choosing values, aspirations, and desires that would give particular meaning to his or her being in the organization. The risks are great.

We propose a new model for being in organizations, a model founded on our beliefs as well as our experiences. I have described the model for our program as "unfolding" and I envision the organizational design of the program as a circle (Boykin, 1990). It is similar to Fox's (1979) description of "dancing Sarah's circle." This is, in fact, the paradigm of the program today. All persons who have a commitment to the teaching and study of nursing are envisioned to be dancers in this open circle. Persons sharing in the dance of nursing might include members of the Board of Regents, the president, the provost, the chief academic officer, the chief financial officer, the vice president of the foundation, the dean of graduate studies and research, the faculty, the students, the dean, the alumni, and the community. Because it is a circle and not a hierarchy, all persons are at the same level. Therefore, there is the opportunity to truly know each other as caring person. Each dancer makes a unique contribution toward accomplishing the program's hopes and dreams. Each dancer is recognized, valued, and celebrated for the gifts he or she brings. No one role is more important than another. Each person's role is valued because, in some way, it supports the accomplishment of program goals and mission. I have found the vision of the common dance to be very empowering. The dancers in the circle come to know each other as caring person and come to appreciate each person's unique role.

A comment on the notion of role is appropriate at this point. All roles are "content-less" unless the focus of the role is made clear. When individuals are in the dance of nursing, each person is there for what he or she can offer to the process of nursing education. This would mean, for example, providing an adequate budget for the college, fund-raising to accomplish particular college goals, and so on. The role influences how the person in the role lives out the commitment to nursing education. Very important to this conceptualization is the assumption that everyone in the circle is committed to the dance of nursing and therefore will participate in securing and providing appropriate resources.

The role of administrator or dean of a caring-based nursing program must be intrinsically linked to an understanding of nursing as a discipline and profession. The administrator of a caring-based nursing program directs all actions toward creating, maintaining, and supporting a caring environment in which knowledge of the discipline can be discovered. The administrator nurtures ideas, secures resources, communicates the nature of the discipline, models living and growing in caring, co-creates a culture in which the study of nursing can be achieved freely and fully, grounds all actions in a commitment to caring as a way of being, and treats others with the same care, concern, and understanding as those entrusted to our nursing care.

As dean, there is an obligation to make sure that *all* actions originate in caring. Moral obligations arise from commitment to the belief that the nature of being human is to be caring and that "a caring environment is one in which all aspects of the human person are respected, nurtured, and celebrated" (Florida Atlantic University philosophy). These beliefs direct ways of relating with administrators, faculty, students, and the community at large.

In all relationships, the challenge of every encounter is to live caring—to be open to knowing caring in that moment. I find the use of alternating rhythms a helpful tool in transforming an encounter to a caring encounter. The concept of alternating rhythms stresses the importance of using narrowing and widening vantage points in order that situations be understood. Greater understanding of persons in their particular roles is gleaned as one attempts to enter that world, gain an additional perspective, and use this knowledge as a way to understand the situation and to witness expressions of caring in that moment.

I would like to share some examples in which the expressed beliefs about caring, person, and nursing directed the action of the dean. These examples come from relationships with administration, fellow colleagues, students, and the community at large. Let me begin with a couple of situations involving administrators:

- To begin a new program of study in the Florida state university system, approval of the Board of Regents is required. The request to initiate another master's degree program in nursing was not approved when first requested. Rather than wait the designated period of time to resubmit the proposal, the dean requested to address a joint meeting of the Board of Regents and the Post-Secondary Education Commission to articulate the program's unique focus and the need for the program in our community. The dean expected administration to support this request because their collective role was to facilitate the accomplishment of program goals. The support was in fact given, and approval was secured.

- Formulas used for budget allocations do not provide adequate funding for high-intensity practice programs of study such as nursing. The need for a broader budget perspective was brought to the Council of Deans. This factor, as well as others, resulted in the creation of a task force to focus on a new model for the budget process. Helping others to understand the discipline and the unique needs of the program will be an ongoing effort. What is significant is the willingness of others to hear the call for greater understanding and to respond to this call. Herein, again, lies support for the assumption that the chief financial officer and others are in their roles to support the individual program needs.

Chapter 5 illustrates that no model is devoid of struggles. It is only through listening and coming to know each other that caring environments are created. The role of dean provides multiple opportunities to relate to faculty in a way that is reflective of expressed values. For example:

- When prospective faculty interview in the College of Nursing, I ask them to share with me their most beautiful story of nursing. This has become a way for me to know the person as both caring person and nurse. It is also a way to know the person's love of and passion for the discipline. An expressed love of nursing is very important to me because I believe this will then be modeled to students.

• When the faculty created the College Promotion and Tenure Guidelines, many divergent views were expressed. This situation required that much time be spent in what seemed to be unending dialogue. This process was necessary in order that all views could be understood and that all Faculty as well as administrators were comfortable with the product.

• In an effort to help us know each other better as person and faculty member, annual retreats are held. Two years ago, the focus of the retreat was *coming to know ourselves as caring and creative persons*. After listening to a guided imagery tape, faculty wrote down a story of nursing practice. This was followed by an opportunity to aesthetically represent the essence of the story. Aesthetic expressions were shared with faculty, and we came to know each other as person and nurse. An example of a faculty expression from this retreat follows:

NURSING

Formless, floating, a cloud of
misty possibility
within and without,
you, me, us . . . all of us . . .
But you and me
connected, connecting
floating together, apart,
creating together the fiber of our
being.
You tell me in so many ways
who you are and how you are.
We are

in a moment and forever
changed from the moment.

I am a staff nurse.
You are wheeled in the door of the
intensive care unit
covered with white sheet . . .
fear in your eyes . . .
body not responding to your
desire, needs, hopes.
Will it ever?
We work so quickly to get you into
the giant iron house that will allow
you to breathe.
I am so busy, so afraid I will do
the wrong thing.
I don't belong here.
I want to flee,
be anywhere but here.

Formless.
A void.
Waiting for the form.
Trying to force it be . . .
and nothing
but my fear.

Your eyes—panic, pleading,
needing, questioning—
Stepping out of self and moving
into the cloud, pulled by your pleading eyes,
creating the form of healing,
caring with you for a moment of
days
into weeks.

A husband, a mother,
part of the mist

brought into the light of our
creating stolen moments
illegal passing through the door
into the healing space.

And one day, by allowing to be,
the body, the whole, the healing
space . . .
You move a toe, and smile, and
speech returns,
and you are wheeled triumphant
from the clanking world of
technology and beeping and never-
ending glaring fluorescent lights.
And I hold your hand and share
your joy as you settle into a new
bed in a new place.
And gradually we break apart,
lose touch.

And months later,
A lifetime of time
and of moments.
I am back into the daily,
the beeping, rustling, bustling,
hurrying,
heart banging world.
And you walk in the door.
I don't know you,
upright, strong, radiant,
come to share the joy of your
becoming, of our creation.

And I know a golden cloud,
warm and rosy haze of the joy of
our connection.

> We embrace,
> say the usual things we say,
> we all say,
> and move out into the pulse beat of
> our lives.
>
> *by Carolyn Brown*

- I have become quite sensitive to the use of the pronoun "my" and try to avoid using expressions such as "my faculty," "my secretary," and "my students." Such phrases, although frequently used, unconsciously language an objectification of other and the uniqueness of person may be lost.

- As dean of a caring-based program, one of the responsibilities is to facilitate the creation of an academic environment that frees faculty and students to live out authentically who they are and supports their continual growth. Faculty may negotiate teaching assignments with each other and, through the process, come to know how colleagues may like to grow. Faculty need to be free to share not only their dreams and goals related to the role of faculty, but they need to be supported in living these out.

The dean assists in creating an environment that fosters the development of the students' capacity to care. These suggestions have proven effective:

- Express a desire to know students as caring persons, invite them to open dialogues with the dean. Frequently, this time is spent sharing stories of nursing practice. Informal dialogue provides an opportunity for students to come to know the dean as person.

- Project an openness and a desire to be available to and for students. Students learn through modeling that respect for person is basic to all interactions. Therefore, although there may clearly be an "open door" policy, students must know that situations involving faculty or other students will not be heard unless all parties are present.
- In all policy formulations and implementations, allow for unique student situations to be considered. Policies exist for exceptions.

The dean is in a unique position to act as liaison with the community. Consumers of health care enhance their commitment and facilitate the securing of resources needed to achieve program excellence when they understand the full meaning of living a caring-based program. In our situation:

- Negotiations between the vice presidents of nursing of several health care agencies in the community and the College of Nursing resulted in the agencies' donating to the College, for between 6 and 12 hours per week, the services of a few expert staff nurses who taught sections of nursing practice courses at their hospitals. The agencies agreed to release these individuals to provide their services at no cost to the College. There was mutual benefit to the agencies. These expert nurses attended 16 hours of orientation in order to understand the philosophy of the College and to study how to teach nursing in a practice setting using a caring-based lens.
- Dialogue with donors from the community resulted in the establishment of a loan forgiveness fund at two local hospitals as well as numerous scholarship funds.

An administrator's competence in living a caring-based program may be evidenced by the extent to which formal and informal aspects of the program convey caring. One must seek to know person as person and to create a freeing environment in which all aspects of the person are respected, nurtured, and celebrated. There must be an appreciation of self and other and an understanding of our interconnectedness. I found it helpful to reflect on these questions in the process of living a caring-based program:

- How do I model caring in my day-to-day living?
- What should the design of a caring-based program look like?
- How can I free myself and others to become and to live out our authentic self?
- How do my actions reflect my commitment to the discipline?
- How can the uniqueness of caring in nursing be articulated?

REFERENCES

Boykin, A. (1990). Creating a caring environment: Moral obligations in the role of dean. In M. Leininger & J. Watson, *The caring imperative in education* (pp. 247–254). New York: National League for Nursing.

Fox, M. (1979). *Spirituality named compassion.* Minneapolis, MN: Winston Press.

Mayeroff, M. (1971). *On caring.* New York: Harper & Row.

Roach, S. (1984). *Caring: The human mode of being. Implications for nursing.* Toronto: Faculty of Nursing, University of Toronto, Perspectives in Caring, Monograph I.

Nursing: A Discipline of Knowledge Grounded in Caring

Marilyn E. Parker

*W*hat values and beliefs of university nursing faculty form the basis for teaching, scholarship, and practice in nursing?

What are the faculty's various approaches to teaching, scholarship, and practice in the discipline of nursing?

What assertions and practices of nursing faculty justify and ensure that nursing as a discipline of knowledge is appropriate for academic study within the university?

In what ways can beliefs about caring in nursing be actualized as the basis for teaching, scholarship, and practice in the discipline of nursing?

Nursing is a discipline of knowledge incorporating an area of study and a field of professional practice. This chapter describes the views held by the faculty of the College of Nursing, Florida Atlantic University (FAU), toward the discipline of nursing. Sources of information for this description are documents prepared by the faculty and included in the Self Study Report (Florida Atlantic University Division of Nursing, 1990) prepared for a National League for Nursing site visit. Some illustrations of how faculty live their beliefs in the teaching and learning of nursing have been taken from examples offered by faculty for this chapter.

Research and publication are essential faculty contributions to the development of the discipline. Publications of faculty scholarship may be reviewed for expressions of faculty thinking and research presented in the nursing literature. Examples of recent citations of faculty scholarship are offered in the following references at the end of this chapter: Beck, 1993a, 1993b; Boykin & Schoenhofer, 1990, 1991, 1993; Coffman, 1992; Coffman, Levitt, & Brown (in press); Cope, 1992; Folden & Coffman, 1993; Locsin, 1993; Parker, 1990, 1993; Ray, 1992; Schoenhofer, 1993; Schuster, 1990, 1992; Tappen & Beckerman, 1992; Winland-Brown & Maheady, 1990; and Winland-Brown & Pohl, 1990.

CHARACTERISTICS OF DISCIPLINE

Conceptions of nursing as a discipline and profession, as held by nursing faculty, encourage a comprehensive perspective on nursing. King and Brownell's classic work (1976) about disciplines of knowledge defined discipline as not only a network of content and an area of study but also a community of scholars sharing a domain of inquiry and a commitment to specific aspects of human affairs. Other attributes of a discipline, as described by these authors, include:

1. An expression of human imagination;
2. A tradition;
3. A syntactical structure;
4. A conceptual structure;
5. A specialized language or system of symbols;
6. A heritage of literature, artifacts, and networks of communications;
7. A valuative and affective stance;
8. An instructive community. (p. 95)

Using these characteristics, interconnections among nurses in practice, education, administration, and research within an inclusive context of discipline and profession are invited and supported. Faculty members of the College of Nursing try to live as a community of scholars committed to developing and using knowledge for purposes of nursing study and practice, and thus endeavor to bring to life nursing as an integrated discipline of knowledge and professional practice.

FOCUSING THE DISCIPLINE OF NURSING

The curriculum as well as the scholarly and practice activities of the faculty are based on the fundamental belief that nursing is a discipline of knowledge and professional practice.

Further, documents of the faculty assert that the discipline of nursing is dependent for its content and organization on a conception of nursing that sets forth a unique focus for nursing. The concepts of nursing held by the nursing faculty define the discipline and practice of nursing, and permit description of what is and is not nursing knowledge and nursing practice. Thus, the goals and boundaries of nursing knowledge and practice are assured and the place of nursing in society is clarified. Beliefs about nursing and about the discipline of knowledge and professional practice are the basis for purposes and processes engaged in by the nursing faculty, and these beliefs anchor the nursing curricula.

The fundamental ideas that direct the ways of being of the College of Nursing faculty and their work of developing conceptual and syntactical structures of the discipline, can be found in the philosophy statement reproduced in Chapter 1. These beliefs include:

1. Caring as the essence of being human;
2. Caring in nursing as the mutual human process in which the nurse artistically responds with authentic presence to a call from the client;
3. Caring in nursing as the basis for examination and further development of the discipline.

Conceptions of persons and nursing held by the faculty assist in understanding the views of the discipline and practice used in the work of the faculty. Person is recognized as a unique individual who has a oneness with others and the environment, connected with them in caring relationships. Further, the faculty, in its statement of philosophy, equates the nature of being human with being caring and being "free for choosing values, aspirations and desires which give meaning to living and reflect well being. Well being is creating and living the meaning of life." The well-being and becoming of individuals, families, groups, communities, and societies are fostered through caring interrelationships with others and with the environment.

The view of person guides relations and actions of the faculty within the College of Nursing and toward the community-at-large. The view of person, along with the conception of nursing, guides thinking about nursing, assuring unique contributions to the discipline in forms of practice, scholarship, teaching, and learning. Building on the view of person, the conception of nursing as promotion of the process of being and becoming through caring sets forth the unique focus of the discipline and practice of nursing. Beliefs about nursing as a discipline of knowledge and professional practice then form the basis for relating with colleagues committed to other bodies of knowledge and areas of service within the larger community.

Following the characteristics of King and Brownell (1976), the discipline of nursing has several requirements to be met and described. The ways in which nursing as a discipline of knowledge and professional practice is characterized will not only define the discipline and practice but will distinguish nursing from other disciplines and practices, eliminating the fuzziness nursing has often tolerated. For example, what is the language of nursing? What symbols, patterns of actions, and ways of viewing person distinguish nursing from other health practices? A survey of the array of nursing books, periodicals, and magazines serves to raise questions about the domain of the discipline and the focus of the practice of nursing and helps in understanding the need for clear alignment with attributes of disciplines of knowledge.

The focus of a discipline states the specific domain of human concern to which the community of scholars must direct attention (King and Brownell, 1976, p. 92). This reason-for-being of each discipline is defined by society-at-large as well as by members of the discipline who are part of that society. The clear focus of the discipline and practice of nursing, as set forth by the faculty, is the promotion of processes of being and becoming through caring. Individuals and groups making up society reflect nursing's domain of human concern by issuing calls for nursing to promote processes of being and becoming through caring. Nurses, in their practice, education, and scholarship, have responded to these calls by defining and developing (1) substantive and syntactical structures of knowledge and practice and (2) forms of education and codes of professional practice that address issues of the domain of human concern.

The place of nursing in the university is a powerful reflection that nursing has a unique focus in society and that nursing scholarship and practice must be clearly guided by this focus in order to survive in the academic community. Nursing has responsibility for specific knowledge and relevant forms of inquiry to further this knowledge. Members of the discipline share the obligation for professional practice in response to society's calls for nursing. Perspectives on nursing as a discipline of knowledge and professional practice set forth the place of nursing within the university, including the broad areas that are of concern within the academic community: faculty, curriculum, students, administration, and governance.

STRUCTURES AND PROCESSES OF THE DISCIPLINE

The conceptual structure of nursing is increasingly rich; the broad range of nursing theories is surveyed and used by students in both undergraduate and graduate courses. The conception of nursing as the promotion of the process of being and becoming through caring is the focus of the structure of the discipline, but this conception does not exclude study and use of other frameworks and theories of nursing. The curriculum accommodates many theories and approaches, being clearly inclusive rather than eclectic. The work of the faculty is grounded in nursing as caring, which permits and encourages study of other conceptual models of nursing.

The syntactical structure of disciplines addresses questions and responses appropriate for study as well as methods of inquiry and ways of teaching and learning in the discipline. Concept and syntax are closely related, and often interconnected, in the nursing programs at Florida Atlantic University. This encourages the ideal experiences of joining teaching, research, and practice in the classroom and clinical learning settings.

Nursing Concepts, Objectives, and Inquiry

Knowledge of the discipline of nursing has been described and formed by nursing faculty for use in the curricula of both the undergraduate and graduate nursing programs. From the fundamental beliefs of faculty, the following five general nursing concepts are organized into a curriculum structure that provides a mode of inquiry for each course:

1. Images of nurse and nursing;
2. Nursing as a discipline of knowledge;
3. Nursing as a profession;
4. Person being and becoming through caring;
5. The practice of nursing.

Each concept is also reflected in purpose statements for curricula of the programs. The concepts are developed into model objectives for each of the nursing courses in the undergraduate and graduate programs. The major concepts and their multiple and extensive interrelationships are introduced early in the curriculum and explored in advancing detail throughout the course of study.

Each objective is broadly stated to invite exploration of the full range of content and learning experiences called for by the complexity of the discipline. Faculty and students may ask themselves, regarding each objective:

What knowledge and experience can be developed in order to achieve this desired outcome?

What nursing practice opportunities in this setting can help develop knowledge in this content area?

What special knowledge and experience, including research, do I bring to the discussion of this objective?

What is the most current nursing and related literature that can inform my exploration of this objective?

This approach for structuring and using objectives based on essential nursing concepts consistently requires inquiry and assurance that the content and learning experiences of each course are continually current. The challenge is to be comfortable with the dynamic processes in teaching and learning that demand constant study and inquiry.

Objectives of the introductory and culminating courses of the undergraduate nursing curriculum and of the first course in the study of advanced practice in the graduate nursing program illustrate the use of the structure of these concepts in the curriculum. (See Table 3–1.)

Nursing Situations and Ways of Knowing

The theory and practice of nursing are vitally connected; classroom and clinical learning experiences are about the knowledge and practice of nursing. Such knowledge and practice are inseparable in the study and doing of nursing. Content and processes for teaching and learning in classroom and clinical areas are derived from study of nursing situations: the lived experiences in which caring between nurse and client fosters well-being. Questions are asked of each nursing situation as knowing of each unique instance of nursing is developed. For example: How is the person in this situation being and becoming through caring? What are calls for nursing to promote caring? What are possible nursing responses? Carper's (1978) ways of knowing in nursing are used as a means of inquiry into nursing situations. (Chapter 4 offers further descriptions of use of nursing situations and the ways of knowing in nursing inquiry.)

Another illustration of the importance of the concept of the nursing situation is in questions posed by graduate nursing students for thesis research. Nursing research addresses questions of the lived experience of caring between nurse and client to promote well-being; and data generation and analysis methods are often from the realm of human science methods of inquiry (Polkinghorn, 1983; Van Manen, 1991). Several nursing faculty are developing methods of inquiry more suited to nursing research questions (see Beck, 1993b; Munhall & Oiler, 1993; Parker, 1994; Parker, Gordon, & Brannon, 1992; Ray, 1991).

Table 3–1

Structure of Major Curriculum Concepts, as Illustrated by Objectives of Three Courses

NUR 3115. Introduction to Nursing as a Discipline and Profession	NUR 4827. Introduction to Professional Nursing	NGR 6941. Introduction to Advanced Nursing Practice: Practicum
1. Develop an appreciation of images of nurse and nursing held, over time, by: a. students of nursing; b. nurses in practice; c. other health care workers; d. society.	1. Express an integrated image of nurse as beginning practitioner in a range of nursing situations, and of nursing as a discipline and profession.	1. Evaluate images of nurse and nursing in advanced nursing practice.
2. Express an understanding of nursing as a discipline of knowledge, including: a. characteristics of disciplines of knowledge; b. ways of knowing fundamental nursing; c. major theoretical conceptions of nursing; d. conception of nursing held by FAU School of Nursing faculty; e. modes of inquiry; f. relationships among disciplines.	2. Demonstrate an integrated understanding of the knowledge of nursing essential for beginning professional practice.	2. Synthesize advanced nursing knowledge and modes of inquiry required for a range of nursing situations.

3. Express an understanding of nursing as a profession, including:
   a. characteristics of a profession and professionhood;
   b. social responsibility and accountability;
   c. personal and professional leadership;
   d. values, standards, ethical and legal systems;
   e. education patterns.

4. Value the meaning of being and becoming through caring as central to understanding person and persons, including:
   a. choosing values, aspirations, and desires;
   b. expressions of caring;
   c. caring relationships with individuals, families, groups, communities, others.

5. Envision nursing as the promotion of the process of being and becoming through caring.

3. Actualize values and standards of professional nursing within a range of nursing situations.

4. Interpret the meaning of being and becoming through caring expressed in calls and responses of person and persons from the perspective of the beginning practitioner of nursing.

5. Demonstrate nursing as the promotion of the process of being and becoming through caring in a range of nursing practice situations.

3. Analyze nursing situations from the perspective of the practitioner of advanced nursing:
   a. professional responsibility and accountability;
   b. values, standards, and ethical, political, and legal issues.

4. Examine the meaning of being and becoming through caring, as understood by clients and nurses in a variety of advanced nursing practice situations.

5. Interpret nursing as the promotion of the process of being and becoming through caring in situations of advanced nursing practice.

Illustrations of Teaching and Learning about Nursing

Teaching and learning experiences focused on nursing situations in many settings include a range of opportunities, with emphasis on students' being very active in the study of nursing. There is probably less lecture and more interaction in this curriculum than in most others. Dialogue is the order of each day. Assignments include reflection and writing about the literature, nursing practice, questions for research, and the development of the individual and unique student of nursing. Students are directed to read primary literature sources; emphasis is on original publications of nursing theory, research, and other scholarship. The nursing situation is always the focus of the study of nursing.

Nursing faculty were invited to provide examples of how nursing as a discipline and practice is studied in classroom and clinical teaching situations. Several of these illustrations are offered here.

1. The first undergraduate course in which students study clinical nursing is titled General Nursing Situations. The cumulative experience of this course is the development and presentation of an "aesthetic project," which provides an opportunity to express a fully integrated understanding of a nursing situation. Students may use any medium of aesthetic expression to represent a nursing situation of their experience. The sense of a lived experience in which the caring between nurse and the one nursed promotes well-being is thus represented and shared in the classroom.

2. One teacher who has students in clinical settings with parents and children asks the students to prepare a weekly clinical analysis paper from a pro forma worksheet. The points considered in the clinical analysis guide the

student in developing and using knowledge of the discipline. Students are asked to identify the personal, empirical, ethical, and aesthetic knowledge they have used to create the caring experiences of nursing. The papers include descriptions of calls for nursing and nursing responses to these calls. Outcomes of the nursing situations are described as examples of how the caring between the nurse and client promotes well-being.

3. One teacher who had students in a hospital setting for clinical learning experiences wrote:

> In the acute care course I teach, students are encouraged/ required to prepare for clinical [experiences] by asking themselves: What do I need to know to adequately promote the process of being and becoming through caring with this unique patient? As students provide care for the patients, they raise and record clinically based questions designed to further their understanding of the nursing situations and begin to build on previous experience. Students reflect on these questions and access the literature in ways that contribute to their understanding as opposed to answering "simple" technical questions. Through the semester, students' understanding of the body of nursing knowledge and the focus of practice is reflected in increasing depth and breadth.

4. From a teacher of an elective course in transcultural nursing came these comments:

> We study nursing as a discipline of knowledge and professional practice by considering relations between transcultural nursing theory and nursing practice with a specific cultural group, and ways persons in this group can be cared for in various practice settings (home, hospital, community, institution). Examples from nursing practice show interdependence of the discipline and

practice of nursing—a tradition, a human caring science, and a commitment to effective living or beliefs.

CONTINUING CHALLENGES

The discipline of nursing is often experienced as a search—a search for the meaning of nursing, for the right questions, and for ways to be better informed and gain fuller knowing about nursing knowledge and practice. The history of the discipline, as told in its structures, traditions, literature, language, and instructive communities, continues as the stories of the faculty of the College of Nursing unfold. Many know nursing as a way of being: everyday experiences tell of nursing as a way of life, a way of living. Nursing can be so absorbing that, in the same way the aspects of the discipline direct work of the faculty, the values and beliefs about nursing as a discipline often guide the day-to-day living of the nurse.

How can the nursing faculty gain the confidence and energy they need to refine the work of the discipline and practice begun at FAU?

How can we have courage to go forward with our work so well begun?

What is the measure of the possibilities of extension and the speed of development of the discipline if nursing faculty maintain commitment to development of nursing knowledge based on a unique focus of nursing as a discipline and practice?

REFERENCES

Beck, C. T. (1993a). Teetering on the edge: A substantive theory of postpartum depression. *Nursing Research, 42*(1), 42–48.

Beck, C. T. (1993b). Qualitative research: The evaluation of its credibility, fittingness and audibility. *Western Journal of Nursing Research, 15*(2), 263–266.

Boykin, A., & Schoenhofer, S. (1990). Caring in nursing: Analysis of extant theory. *Nursing Science Quarterly, 3*(2), 149–155.

Boykin, A., & Schoenhofer, S. (1991). Story as link between nursing practice, ontology, epistemology. *Image: The Journal of Nursing Scholarship, 23*(4), 245–248.

Boykin, A., & Schoenhofer, S. (1993). *Nursing as caring: A model for transforming nursing practice.* New York: National League for Nursing.

Carper, B. (1978). Fundamental patterns of knowing in nursing. *Advances in Nursing Science, 1*(1), 13–23.

Coffman, S. (1992). Home care of the child and family after near drowning. *Journal of Pediatric Health Care, 6*(1), 18–24.

Coffman, S., Levitt, M. & Brown, L. (in press). Clarification of expectations in prenatal couples: Contribution to postbirth outcomes. *Nursing Research.*

Cope, D. (1992). Self-esteem and the practice of breast self-examination. *Western Journal of Nursing Research, 14*(5), 618–631.

Florida Atlantic University Division of Nursing. (1990). *Self study report,* Boca Raton: The University.

Folden, S., & Coffman, S. (1993). Respite care for families of children with disabilities. *Journal of Pediatric Health Care, 7*(3), 103–110.

King, A., & Brownell, J. (1976). *The curriculum and the disciplines of knowledge.* Huntington, NY: Krieger.

Locsin, R. C. (1993). Time experiences among selected institutionalized older clients. *Clinical Nursing Research, 2*(4), 451–463.

Munhall, P. L., & Oiler, C. J. (1993). *Nursing research: A qualitative perspective.* New York: National League for Nursing.

Parker, M. E. (Ed.). (1990). *Nursing theories in practice.* New York: National League for Nursing.

Parker, M. E. (Ed.). (1993). *Patterns of nursing theories in practice.* New York: National League for Nursing.

Parker, M. E. (1994). Living nursing values in nursing practice. In D. A. Gaut & A. Boykin (Eds.), *Caring as healing: Renewal through hope.* New York: National League for Nursing.

Parker, M. E., Gordon, S. C., & Brannon, P. (1992). Involving nursing staff in research: a non-traditional approach. *Journal of Nursing Administration, 22*(4), 58–63.

Polkinghorn, D. (1983). *Methodology for the human sciences: Systems of inquiry.* Albany: SUNY Press.

Ray, M. (1991). Caring inquiry: The aesthetic process in the way of compassion. In D. A. Gaut & M. M. Leininger (Eds.), *Caring: The compassionate healer.* New York: National League for Nursing.

Ray, M. (1992). Critical theory as a framework to enhance nursing science. *Nursing Science Quarterly, 5*(3), 98–101.

Schoenhofer, S. (1993). What constitutes nursing research? *Nursing Science Quarterly, 6*(2), 5–6.

Schuster, E. A. (1990). Earth caring. *Advances in Nursing Science, 13*(1), 25–30.

Schuster, E. A. (1992). Earth dwelling. *Holistic Nursing Practice, 6*(4), 1–9.

Tappen, R., & Beckerman, A. (1992). Hospitalization of the frail older adult. *Geriatric Nursing, 13*(2), 149–152.

Van Manen, M. (1991). *Researching lived experience.* Ithaca, NY: SUNY Press.

Winland-Brown, J., & Maheady, D. (1990). Using intuition to define homesickness at summer camp. *Journal of Pediatric Health Care, 4*(3), 117–121.

Winland-Brown, J., & Pohl, J. (1990). Administrators' attitudes toward hiring disabled nurses. *Journal of Nursing Administration. 20*(4), 24–27.

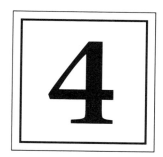

The Shared Study of Nursing

Diane Cope and Marilyn E. Parker

*I*n this chapter, the shared study of nursing (commonly called the curriculum) is discussed. It is our belief that faculty and students co-participate in this study. Teaching and learning occur through open dialogue rather than in a lecture format where facts and principles are disseminated. Implicit in this approach is not only humility, in the recognition that we continually learn from each other, but also a sense of collegiality. Sharing our common love and passion for the discipline is important to understanding what it means to be members of a discipline.

The study of nursing is approached in a nontraditional way through the use of nursing situations. As defined in the philosophy, a nursing situation is "a lived experience in which the caring between nurse and client fosters well-being" (creating and living the meaning of life). Nursing situations have simultaneous commonality and uniqueness. In each nursing situation, there is a call from the client and a response from the nurse. The understanding of the call arises from the nurse's understanding of the uniqueness of the person. Through authentic presence, as caring person, the nurse is able to enter the world of the other, hear calls for nursing, and respond appropriately to promote the process of being and becoming through caring. Inquiry into nursing situations facilitates student understanding of nursing as a discipline of knowledge and professional practice centered in caring.

This study begins in the first required nursing prerequisite course, Introduction to Nursing as a Discipline and Profession. In this course, students are introduced to nursing as a distinct discipline of knowledge and a unique professional practice. Concepts introduced in this course are foundational to the program, comprise the organizing framework, and introduce the themes that are developed into model objectives for each course throughout the undergraduate and graduate programs. The five concepts are: (1) images of nurse and nursing; (2) nursing as a discipline of knowledge; (3) nursing as a profession; (4) person being and becoming through caring; and (5) nursing as the promotion of the process of being and becoming through caring.

In this foundational course, students come to know these concepts through inquiry into the structures and processes of the discipline; exploration and description of what is and is not nursing knowledge and nursing practice; and examination of caring ingredients (knowing, alternating rhythms, patience, honesty, trust, humility, hope, and courage) (Mayeroff, 1971) and caring attributes (conscience, commitment, competence, compassion, and confidence) (Roach, 1987). Students are challenged to know self and other as caring person, to identify calls for nursing, and to envision nursing responses actualizing the ability to care.

Students' understanding of this nursing focus provides a structure for advanced study in subsequent nursing practice courses as they build on the concepts studied in the introductory course. Further, this beginning understanding of nursing as the promotion of the process of being and becoming through caring is the ground of all further nursing development.

Nursing situations are clustered within courses based on traditional and social expectations as well as unfolding possibilities. Therefore, particular situations from a common setting are grouped by course. For example, in the first nursing practice course, students are provided the opportunity to study the meaning of caring as related to self and other in the context of nursing situations involving healthy persons across the life span. In successive nursing practice courses, students study the art of caring in nursing situations involving individuals, families, groups, and communities in a variety of settings, including long-term and acute. In the culminating undergraduate course, Introduction to Professional Nursing Practice, students study nursing situations within organizational structures as caring environments that influence the process of being and becoming for clients, self, colleagues, and the organization. A complete list of course descriptions is presented in Appendix B. Program purpose and objectives are stated in Appendices C (undergraduate) and D (graduate).

Carper's (1978) patterns of knowing constitute a useful framework for organizing the study of nursing in our curriculum. First, these patterns will be briefly described. This description will be followed by an illustration of how the patterns could be used to study a nursing situation.

PATTERNS OF KNOWING

The patterns of knowing are: personal, empirical, ethical, and esthetic.

- Personal knowing is concerned with encountering and actualizing self. Through the actualization of an authentic personal relationship, the nurse accepts others in their freedom to create their own self in their process of becoming.

- Empirical knowing is concerned with the science of nursing and includes general laws and theoretical formulations from nursing and related disciplines. The nurse draws, from a broad knowledge base, the relevant data necessary to understand a particular nursing situation.

- Ethical knowing addresses matters of obligation—what ought to be done. In this program, students explore obligations resulting from a commitment to caring as a way of being.

- Esthetic knowing, which is the art of nursing, integrates the other patterns of knowing in a caring moment. Moving beyond language, the nurse experiences the wholeness of the nursing situation, self, and other in meaningful relationships, and artistically creates unique approaches to care based on the dreams and goals of other within the specific nursing situation.

Each fundamental pattern of knowing subsumes particular kinds of information, although the patterns are not mutually exclusive and one way of knowing does not diminish the importance of other ways of knowing. Through interrelationships and interdependence, each of these patterns comes into play in a nursing situation and guides understanding of the "whole" with caring as the unifying concept.

Because of the nontraditional nature of this approach, questions concerning the process for teaching and learning will naturally present themselves. The illustration and discussion of a nursing situation in the next section may assist in gaining an understanding of this approach.

NURSING SITUATION

AVE MARIA AND THERAPEUTIC TOUCH FOR DAVID

David, let me know your pain;
From fractured leg and heart,
Share with me your private hell.
Next to one who's far,
Far away in his own world;
Moaning, crying, weak.
What's it like to lie beside
One who cannot speak?
Tell me David, what you do
To cancel out the sound;
Eliminate the smell of dung
In which your roommate's found?
Who can you complain about?
Are you worse off than he?
Tied to IV, traction lines
You cannot be free.
David, I can see your pain.
Tell me where you are.

Tied in bed. Powerless.
From loved ones you're apart.
I can't move you from this place
To take your pain away.
But let me lay my hands on you
And sing to you today.

Ave Maria, gratia plena
Maria, gratia plena
Ave dominus, dominus tecum.
Benedicta tu in mulieribus.
Et benedictus
Et benedictus, fructus ventris;
Ventris tui, Jesu.
Ave Maria.

I sang the song he loved and used
To meditate and flee,
Escape tormenting stimuli.
He needed to be freed,
To understand why he must bear
This trial, this hell, this pain,
I sang the tune; I touched with care
To give him peace again.

by Michele Stobie

Michele responded beautifully to David's call for comfort. Through authentic presence, she came to know him in his uniqueness as caring person. Michele's caring response of nursing arose from the call she heard from David to help him discover his freedom, transcending for the moment his pain. Michele artistically responded through song and touch. Another nurse in the same situation may have responded differently, depending on the uniqueness of person brought to the situation. Embedded in each nursing situation is a range of calls and possible nursing responses in the caring moment.

Through the study of nursing situations in the classroom setting, faculty and students, as caring persons, enter into the situation with nurse and person-being-nursed, bringing forth the uniqueness of person. Calls for nursing are identified, and responses to the calls are shared based on the uniqueness of their being. Responses vary and all are correct. Each person risks unveiling self throughout this dialogue.

Following is an analysis of how Carper's patterns of knowing might be used as a framework for study of the nursing situation centered on David. Selected examples of personal knowing that could be brought to the study of nursing include:

1. Students and faculty reflect on who they are as caring person and nurse in this situation;
2. Students ask who is David as caring person and use Mayeroff's caring ingredients as one way to discover this knowledge;
3. There is dialogue on understanding:
   a. the meaning of music to Michele (the nurse) and David (the client);
   b. the meaning of isolation and comfort;
   c. the meaning of being authentically present as caring nurse.

Students select, from a vast repertoire, the empirical knowledge that is needed to understand a particular situation. To be knowledgeable about David's situation, for example, the student would need:

1. To understand the pathophysiology of pain, and traditional and nontraditional ways of alleviating discomfort;

2. To understand, through reading and research, the experience of being isolated and dependent;

3. To know the research that has studied the effect of therapeutic touch and music on pain.

Ethical knowing was called for in several ways:

1. Michele's comfort in taking risks, in having the courage to live out fully her beauty and uniqueness in practice, and in living her personhood through professionhood;

2. David's risk taking, in exposing who he is as person;

3. Michele's commitment to caring, which grounded her response to David.

By integrating each of these patterns, Michele created esthetically a beautiful and unique response to David's call for promoting his being and becoming through caring in the moment.

As can be seen through this example, this is a different way to approach the study of nursing. Faculty foster understanding of nursing situations by posing certain questions grounded in the concept of caring. These broad questions are:

1. Who is this person as caring person?

2. What are the unique hopes and dreams for being and becoming through caring?

3. What are the person's unique calls for nursing?

4. What are the ranges of calls for nursing through this situation?

5. What are the specific nursing responses of caring that may promote the processes of being and becoming through caring?

6. What are the possibilities and the hoped-for outcomes in the nursing situation?

As mentioned earlier, faculty and students co-participate in the study of nursing; their sharing of knowledge and expertise adds to the fullness of the knowledge gleaned. Although there are commonalities in nursing situations, students learn quickly that each situation is unique and expresses its own beauty. Situations studied in class represent the actual lived experiences of students and nurses in nursing practice settings.

Faculty choose settings for practice courses that foster the study of nursing by offering an environment that supports person coming to know self and other as caring persons—an environment in which the beliefs of the program can be lived. In the practice courses, the study of nursing focuses on a range of nursing situations that might apply in particular settings. Prior to engaging in the care of clients, students use centering strategies to focus themselves in preparation for entering nursing situations. Learning to be authentically present in practice is a skill that grows in competence over time. The primary focus of the study of nursing in practice settings occurs most fully in postconferences, which give students the opportunity to bring forth their own nursing situations for study with colleagues. Together, they engage in dialogue about how, as unique individuals, they may have responded to the calls for nursing.

Nursing Situations: Application

We now offer examples of aesthetic expressions of nursing situations, created by undergraduate and graduate students. One example is cited for each nursing practice course in the curriculum that can be used to focus the study of nursing.

NUR 3116L: General Nursing Situations. This first under-graduate nursing practice course has as its purpose facilitating a beginning grasp of the general nature of nursing situations.

TOGETHER FOR A MOMENT IN TIME

Sitting there serenely like a statue
it was as if she had always been there
motionless in time.
A cold room, strange, sad, and sweet faces
one melting into another—all seemed separate,
yet all became one.
I touched her—she pulled away.
We spoke of simple things,
Of our names and our claim to the place of our presence.
It was rocky—I wanted,
she wanted not.
Or so I thought.
The rhythm of the day led into song
and we rose to the occasion.
Suddenly, filled with emotion and glistening eyes she
embraced me.
We were alone together for a moment in time.
Her call, so elusive to me before,
resonated in my being.
She was free to me and I was free from myself to be.
She spoke of loneliness and emptiness
Of darkness and solitude
And anger.
Every day was the same—the same place, same table,
same chairs.
The sameness seemed to envelop her.
Her essence seemed to be lost deep within her.
But our talk and touch moved it up and out.
I knew her and she knew me.
And over the days that we talked, touched, played,

and sat in silence, we entered a unique place together.
We felt anger, isolation, sadness,
warmth, and hope together.
It was with ambivalence that I said goodbye.
As much as I wanted to leave, I wanted to stay.
As I left the room, though, I turned to see that she once again
appeared like a statue sitting
motionless in time.

by Carol Bruce

NUR 3745L: Nursing Situations in Acute Settings: Parents and Children. This course focuses on the study of a range of nursing situations involving parents and children in acute health care settings. Events occurring in this range of situations include pregnancy, childbirth, and children with health alterations requiring care in acute settings.

BORN TOO SOON

Born too soon
I lay in this artificial womb you've created
and wait for your touch.
I feel like broken glass as I lay here
surrounded by the sound of the machines I need.
The flashing light keeps me company as I wait for you.
I sleep as life-giving fluids drip in my veins
and still I wait.
I live for your touch. That's when I feel most alive!
Are you my mother?
I don't know but I love you and know that love
is returned a hundred times
as we rejoice in my progress towards life.
And every day I know that you will come and give me
your loving touch.
And when you come you touch me ever so gently, careful
so as not to dislodge the many tubes that keep me alive.

But they are nothing compared to your touch.
You hold me so softly in your hands—turning me, weighing me,
washing me, recording my progress.
And finally the moment I long for comes as you
hold my hand in yours
stroke my head
and sing a lullaby.

by Elizabeth Dodge

NUR 4746L: Nursing Situations in Acute Settings: Adult. This course focuses on a range of nursing situations that is similar to the range typically seen in what are often called medical–surgical courses.

INTENSIVE CARE

Did you see, nurse, that you can know me—
The part that is me, my mind and soul, is in my eyes.
These tubes that are everywhere—that is not me.
The one in my throat is the worst of all—
Now my whole being, the essence of me, I must reflect
through my hands but they are tied down,
movement of my head but did you realize that is
uncomfortable for me
or through my eyes and you do not notice them—
except once today during my bath.
You speak to me and look at the tubes—
Don't you know my thoughts are all over my face
Don't you realize your thoughts are on your face—
In your touch and your tone of voice.
I wrote a request on paper; you said "I'll take care
of it for you"—your tone said "Why can't this woman
Do anything for herself?"
You positioned your hand to count my pulse but I
Can't say you touched me—you wouldn't hold my
hand that I may touch you.

The Shared Study of Nursing

You walked in for the first time today with a grin
on your face but your mouth is now tight and
You grimaced a lot as you bathed me.
Don't you see, nurse, that you can know me—I'm not
a chart or tubes of medication, monitors or all
the other things you look at so intensely—I'm
more than that—
I'm scared—just look in my eyes.

by Sheila Carr

NUR 4635L: Nursing Situations in the Community: Families/
Groups. This course focuses on diverse nursing situations set
in the community, in the context of families and groups.
There is some emphasis on community health centers as settings for nursing situations.

DIVERSITY

Different customs, different times
People come from varying climes.
What's important in their lives?
Sons and daughters, husbands and wives.
Ways of worship, foods they eat
Rest and hygiene are needs to meet,
How do I communicate?
A smile, a nod, a touch will state.
Though not the same as you or me,
We all share in our need to be.

by Barbara Sorbello

NUR 4747L: Nursing Situations in Home and Rehabilitation
Settings. The range of nursing situations organized within this
course are those set in rehabilitation and long-term centers
and in the home.

TOGETHER, WE BEGIN

I entered your room, to meet you,
hoping to enter your world
to know you.
I am still new at this and certainly
must look as unsure as I feel . . .
but you do not seem to notice.
You are busy . . .
noticing yourself
and this situation
you find yourself in.
You look up, and I see in your eyes
a light of recognition.
You see me as someone who has
come to help you understand
and make sense of this "stroke,"
of this thing that has happened
to you.
So, together we begin to get ready
for the day.
As I comb your hair, you notice
a button
missing from your blouse,
and you are embarrassed.
I am sorry I didn't notice before,
so I adjust things
so no one will see,
and I realize this makes
you feel better.
I check your "tubes," your "sites,"
your vital signs and I
wonder what you feel
and I ask you,
"What do you need?"
Your paralyzed face turns to me,
and cracks a smile.

56

You accept me
and I see that I
will be okay with this,
and that you are, too.

by Diane Zried

NUR 4827L: Introduction to Professional Nursing Practice. The focus of this course is on the movement from student role to that of beginning practitioner of professional nursing. The context of study is that of a specific group of nursing situations and the organizational environment within which nursing is created.

THE CARING SENSE

You see me blossom in your care
The loving caring action that speaks in all languages.
Our eyes meet and we are one in spirit and soul . . .
You hear my cry, whether silent or loud.
And you are there to lift spirits, courage
and to be proud,
For we have shared our interconnecting hands . . .
You smell the many fragrances
of our mixed bouquet.
The hours, the days, the weeks and still you stay
For we have soldered our relationship
forever and a day . . .
You feel many moods,
some soft, some hard.
You feel my skin, my bones, my soul
As we share the secrets never to be told . . .

by Patricia Dittman

NGR 6940: Advanced Nursing: Adult Practicum. This course focuses on an application of advanced nursing and supporting knowledge in nursing practice with adults.

SHE IS STILL BEAUTIFUL

Miss Margaret opened her weary eyes. Lids heavy with pain, tired from months of suffering. Chemotherapy . .,. . Radiation . . . . Can't eat . . . . Can't sleep . . . . Can't walk any more. Her once beautiful face, glowing skin, strong body, has been ravaged by disease. But she is still beautiful.

I could see that she was being well cared for. Miss Margaret was clean, linens fresh, environment safe, I.V. running well, tube feeding intact, foley bag dependent, dressings clean and dry. What else could she need? I knew what I could do for her. We held hands and then I brushed her hair. Stroke after stroke, her soft downy hairs fluttered through the brush. I brushed gently, in a comforting rhythm. How important touch and physical comfort is. As I cared for her, I remembered my mother brushing my hair, and how special and cared for it made me feel. I am glad that Miss Margaret and I shared this moment. We both felt a time of peace and comfort.

Yes, she is still beautiful.

by Barbara Sorbello

NGR 6941: Introduction to Advanced Nursing Practice: Practicum. This course focuses on application of advanced nursing knowledge of caring, research, nursing theory, and leadership in general nursing situations.

BECAUSE I CARE . . .

Because I Care, I bring
    hope to your hopelessness,
Because I care, I see you
    as loving woman and mother

Because I care, I enter
    your world with humility and respect
I honor your belief that
    somehow I can help.
I live your caring with you,
    to cry when sad
    to howl with delight.
Because I care, I want to
    be there with you and for you
    in sharing your pain and joy.

Because you care, I can
    care with you
Caring crates meaning for you and I.

by Daniel L. Little

NGR 6942: Advanced Nursing: Family Practicum. This course focuses on an application of advanced nursing and supporting knowledge in nursing practice with families.

A PRIVATE PLACE

I've weighed the child
And measured him from head to toe
Encrypted terse details of his
    fragility
In jet black ink upon a bureaucratic
    form.
With trailing tubes we move across
to quietly sit together as I finish
    up.
I cannot reach her, cannot see the
    shapes
She sees through vacant, staring
    eyes . . .
Can't know what hopes she had or has.

If I could split this thing
   apart
Then rip it into minute bits and
   fling
Them banished to the howling
   wind
I would begin again . . .
Create it all afresh, entire.
Would grab her in my arms
Across the thrashings of her
   lusty child.

I finish with my work.
She stands encumbered by entangled
   cords
And cannot grasp the plastic bag
To which her dying child is tied.
It is too much for her to bear.

I—helpless—ask naively, "Can I
   help?"
But now somehow she has it gathered
   in.
Without response she moves away,
Unseeing eyes transfixed by inward
   prescience
of Surcease in a far-off, private
   place.

by Sanford M. Russell

NGR 6943: Advanced Nursing: Nursing Administration Practicum. This course focuses on an application of advanced nursing and supporting knowledge in the practice of nursing administration.

TO BE AND BECOME

To be and become is an altered way of living
Giving to give is to touch
To be is to be with you
Only you know what it is to be
The way of life is to live
Yet is it a mirror or is it truth

The reflection is staring us in the face (mirror)
What do you see—is it the reflection of truth
    or lies
Being and becoming is a way of life
To respect one is to respect all
Can you face yourself—
    or is it the face
        The face of a different man
Can you open your heart
    Let the beauty come in
And the client/nurse reflect—see how the mirror
        looks back
    What do the images state
      what will it say
        To be inside
          To grow
            To allow one to be true

These images are there, but only you see them
    The client is there, and is asking
      The arms are outstretched—
        Will you be there to pick up the arms
        Or will they just dangle

Do we have a choice—
    The nurse is there to listen
      To allow the client to be themselves
        Whatever that may be

As the images come together, the shadow of the
past, present, and future joins as one
The client is able to see the beauty inside themselves
   And around them. Is that beauty for that person
     (Alone)

The nurse is offering and choosing,
The harmony and holding—able to see that beauty—
To reach—to hold—
What ever that may be—
   The mind, body, and soul are one
Will you become one—

by Robin Glance

The shared study of nursing is exciting! Unlike a traditional curriculum, the use of situations to study nursing allows for the continual discovery of nursing knowledge. Faculty are not expected to "have all the answers." Students and faculty bring their breadth and depth of knowledge and experience to this study and learn from and with each other. Together they dance the dance of nursing.

REFERENCES

Bruce, C. (1993). Together for a moment in time. *Nightingale Songs, 2*(1). P.O. Box 057563, West Palm Beach, FL 33405-7563.

Carper, B. (1978). Fundamental patterns of knowing. *Advances in Nursing Science, 1*(1), 13–23.

Carr, S. (1991). Intensive care. *Nightingale Songs, 2*(1). P.O. Box 057563, West Palm Beach, FL 33405-7563.

Dittman, P. (1991). The caring sense. *Nightingale Songs, 1*(3). P.O. Box 057563, West Palm Beach, FL 33405-7563.

Dodge, E. (1992). Born too soon. *Nightingale Songs, 2*(2). P.O. Box 057563, West Palm Beach, FL 33405-7563.

Glance, R. (1991). To be and become. *Nightingale Songs, 2*(1). P.O. Box 057563, West Palm Beach, FL 33405-7563.

Little, D. (1992). Because I care. *Nightingale Songs, 2*(3). P.O. Box 057563, West Palm Beach, FL 33405-7563.

Mayeroff, M. (1971). *On caring.* New York: Harper & Row.

Roach, Sr. S. (1987). *The human act of caring.* Canadian Hospital Association.

Russell, S. (1990). A private place. *Nightingale Songs, 1*(2). P.O. Box 057563, West Palm Beach, FL 33405-7563.

Sorbello, B. (1992). She is still beautiful. *Nightingale Songs, 2*(3). P.O. Box 057563, West Palm Beach, FL 33405-7563.

Sorbello, B. (1992). Diversity. *Nightingale Songs, 2*(3). P.O. Box 057563, West Palm Beach, FL 33405-7563.

Stobie, M. (1991). Ave Maria and therapeutic touch for David. *Nightingale Songs, 1*(3). P.O. Box 057563, West Palm Beach, FL 33405-7563.

Zried, D. (1992). Together, we begin. *Nightingale Songs, 2*(2). P.O. Box 057563, West Palm Beach, FL 33405-7563.

The Experience of Struggle, Freedom, and Growth

Sherrilyn Coffman and
Rozzano C. Locsin

What is the meaning of being a faculty member or professional staff person responsible for bringing a new curriculum to life? This chapter offers descriptions of the struggles and satisfactions involved, from the personal points of view of nursing faculty and professional staff of the Florida Atlantic University College of Nursing. The struggles reflect individual efforts to learn how to be with one another and with students, the responsibilities of living out the caring philosophy, and the ongoing decisions required for creating a nursing curriculum. As they struggle to create a new way of being, faculty and staff describe the satisfactions that emerge: feelings of connectedness, support for one another, and respect, as well as personal freedom, a sense of wholeness, and growth.

The data for this chapter came from 13 (of 19) members of the faculty, and 2 professional staff persons ($n = 15$). Faculty and staff were asked to respond in writing to this question:

> What is the meaning for you of being a member of the Florida Atlantic University College of Nursing faculty and professional staff group?

Three faculty members did independent content analysis of the written data presented, identifying themes. They then met, compared results, and arrived at consensus about the themes. Analysis revealed themes of struggle, being stuck, respect, support, connectedness, wholeness, freedom, and growth. Themes were interrelated, with meaning segments of data often reflecting more than one theme. Three overarching themes emerged: (1) struggle, (2) support, and (3) growth. These themes form the organizing framework for this chapter.

STRUGGLE

The struggle of being a member is one theme that emerged from the faculty and staff members' descriptions of what it means to be a part of the College of Nursing. This theme was described in several ways: striving to know (what it is like, what it takes to be); struggling to conspire, to participate in the unfolding, and to confirm, with patience or impatience, what nursing is as a discipline and a profession through caring; struggling to be human; and unfolding to become through caring.

Being a member of a cadre of faculty in a dynamic, emerging program in which faculty continually strive for better knowledge of nursing as a discipline and profession was characterized as a struggle to know. One faculty member stated:

> I am at the very early stage of being a member of FAU's College of Nursing—so early that I do not yet experience "membership" in my person, but rather, through assigned responsibilities (role), and some initial activities. It is, at this point, an activity or role-based experience, consumed with basic orientational activities: getting to know who the other members are, how things are done, what things mean, and so on, and noting possibilities in the situation. Through discernment of possibilities, I will begin to fashion a way of being a member of the faculty that could be beneficial to me personally, and to the College.

With an emphasis on caring in the curriculum, faculty noted greater awareness of what the responsibility for caring with each other really means. "Coming to awareness" was described as observing these activities: "How faculty greet each other, how faculty compete in a model that fosters cooperation, for example, how faculty work out conflicts between system functions and nurturing activities." The importance of achieving balance as one struggles to become a member of the faculty group was described: "I try to communicate, to make sure my perceptions and what I see or experience are in some type of balance."

In designing a curriculum around caring, the challenge is to maintain consistency about the meaning of the concept of caring. One faculty member noted that caring is often misconstrued as "being nice to each other all the time." The difficulty of expressing negative emotions was described:

> To some extent, we have allowed our valuing of each other as persons to get in the way of progress. It is difficult to have great respect and confidence in someone and question the value of his or her actions at the same time. It is also difficult to teach about "caring for others" in a nurse–client context, where patients' views are seldom countered and positive affect is valued, and then act in a way that is interpreted as negative in faculty relations.

The frustration in the struggle to maintain the expression of faculty or staff member as person, professional, and participant in the faculty group, with responsibilities that influence the emergence of the program, was also noted. Maintaining the identity of person in the group was as important as knowing what this "membership" means to the individual. One staff member, a registered nurse who works in the campus learning laboratory, described this "struggle" to know:

> The students aren't aware of the difference in my role . . . and sometimes the faculty aren't real clear either, and this causes me tension and stress because I find I am continually clarifying my role for both groups.

Another professional staff person described her role as somewhat stressful:

> Because I am a professional nurse, I am interested in the growth of my profession, and yet I am not part of the faculty who decide what the teaching about the profession will look like here at FAU. I express my thoughts mostly in informal ways rather than in formal settings with faculty.

Thus, the struggle to communicate is influenced by role in the College.

The struggle to conspire, to participate in the unfolding, and to confirm nursing as a discipline and a profession through caring is endured with active patience. One individual expressed the meaning of being a faculty member as:

> . . . exercising a great deal of patience, struggling to keep humility front and center, gratitude for the patience and hard work of others, alternating between hopefulness and struggling to keep hope alive in nursing being established as an academic discipline and a learned profession.

The struggle to describe the meaning of being a faculty member was portrayed as striving to know what it is to be human. "Exasperation" and "challenge" were words used by one faculty member. These words increased the need to know more about what it is to be a "challenged" faculty member in the College of Nursing. One individual described her experiences:

> The "exasperation" is probably a natural extension of the turning inward that we have had to do to revise our policies and procedures. My exasperation focuses on the issue of clinical teaching/learning. I haven't agreed with some of the changes that we have made in clinical experiences. I have always made my opinions clearly known, but sometimes I have felt that my opinions were not given due consideration, in the name of expediency. At times I have felt very alone in this struggle.

The struggle to be a part of the whole and yet be oneself was expressed in others' descriptions. When the expectation of conformity was perceived as stronger than respect for diverse opinion, faculty felt "stuck" in conflict and dissatisfaction. The need to provide a forum in which diversity would be recognized and dealt with was pointed out by one faculty member:

> Only because I persisted in expressing my opinions have I been listened to. To some extent, there is still strength in numbers on this faculty, and we need to work, as a group, in better consideration of minority opinions. It is perhaps because I have such high expectations of our group that I feel this way.

Another person noted the importance of recognizing diversity: "One of the issues that we are working on right now as a faculty group is allowing expression of a wide range of ideas, both 'positive' and 'negative' points, and seeing that as necessary."

"Can differences be included without losing the value of the shared vision?" asked another faculty member. A member asked: "Can the vision change? How and with whom should the changing of vision occur?"

Struggling to be human, and unfolding to become through caring, was described by one member of the College of Nursing faculty as an experience that ". . . requires [us] to acknowledge our humanness and to have courage to be open and honest with each other." Yet, these struggles of "seeing the caring in the moment" have been helpful "to better know and respect the other as person."

SUPPORT

The second major theme, support, grew out of subthemes of connectedness and respect. Although respect for one another sometimes emerged through struggle, a sense of connectedness (related to shared interests) also contributed to respect. Respect was just one aspect of a general supportiveness felt by group members.

Their special sense of connectedness was greatly valued by faculty members, one of whom described the feeling of being part of a family:

> I possess a sense of belonging and I experience a special connectedness which I share with no one else. This group has become a family to me like I have never known. I believe that some of this meaning comes from my love for nursing and the opportunity to be with others who share in this interest. However, the majority can be attributed to each unique person. There are many qualities which radiate in this group: caring, respect for others, support, encouragement, confidence, warmth, kindness, tears, and laughter.

Connectedness was described on several levels. This same faculty person additionally stated:

> Although the above qualities may only focus on emotional aspects of being with one another, there is much more. Besides the emotional, there is a cognitive aspect that I experience with this group. This group provides a challenge for my thoughts and perceptions.

Concern for the faculty/staff group involved both giving and taking. However, an overriding concern for the group was expressed:

> I am confident that I could call on any one of the group for ideas or reflection or assistance. My ability to be of service to the larger group has been called forth, which I specifically acknowledge and attend to. I truly CARE

what happens to us as a collective, as well as caring for myself individually.

This sense of group connectedness was described by one member as being part of a community:

> I have been reading about community, and all that a true community entails. And I have come closer to obtaining community than in any other group I have been a part of. There is a spirit in this group of faculty that is bigger than we are. The composite of our hopes and dreams truly makes us an entity where the whole is larger than the sum of its parts. In the name of that spirit, I am friends with other persons (faculty) whose strengths attract me, and whose weaknesses (the characteristics that I don't find attractive) become unimportant.

Support and connectedness often go hand-in-hand as two inseparable concepts. One individual described the help that she gains by watching other faculty:

> Seeing other faculty putting multiple roles in play is really important for me—I know I can go to them and say, "How do you do that? Help me with this," and I know I won't be turned away. There is always someone to turn to for help or suggestions so that you never feel that you're all alone.

A faculty member contrasted her experiences at Florida Atlantic University with faculty membership at other universities:

> In other universities where I have worked, the faculty were more self-centered and tended to be envious of other faculty members' achievements—publishing an article, and so on. Here in the College of Nursing, faculty

are truly excited about and share in another faculty member's accomplishments. Faculty are eager to help other faculty members progress. I have had fellow faculty put calls for abstracts, which they thought were relevant to my research, in my mailbox.

Feeling respected and supported was described in other ways: "being cared for"; "being respected as person"; "being listened to regardless of how stupid my questions are or how diverse my viewpoint is"; "being able to argue about a concern in a faculty meeting and walk out arm-in-arm, leaving the discussion behind, knowing that the discussion wasn't toward persons but for the betterment of the curriculum."

GROWTH

Many faculty and staff expressed themes of wholeness, freedom, and growth as characteristic of their experiences. These themes were described as personal attributes, but they were also related to group membership, to "what happens to us as a collective."

The faculty/professional staff group was often described as the background against which individual wholeness and growth were nurtured. When asked to describe the meaning of being a member of the faculty/professional staff group, one individual responded:

For me, the meaning revolves around the concept of being part of a structure that has no boundaries in its ability and desire to nurture, motivate, nourish, and stimulate the mind, body, and soul.

In this structure, I have had the experience of getting to know the other in a way that has enhanced my

73

personal development and growth. There have been op- portunities for sharing of self in an environment that conveyed that there are moments when we each need to and must, if [we prize] the integrity of the structure, be a whole within the total picture, aiming for a fuller under- standing of who we are and why we are here. I have never felt so at home within myself and my profession; there is a harmony and peace in my person.

Another faculty person further described this view of group as structure:

The meaning for me revolves around a concept of struc- ture, of which I have a part, whose boundaries are open and free-flowing. There is freedom of contact, of thought, of reactions and interactions, all of which have enabled me to be me, seeking out opportunities for growth and development within the philosophy of the program. Support, encouragement, and motivation are all parts of this meaning, enabling this growth to be nurtured and exist.

Freedom to be oneself was further described as the "op- portunity to live out authentically who I am as person and col- league": "The opportunity to be and become who I am, not the 'look as if' to fit someone's idea of what one should 'be' here." Within this free environment, risk taking is possible. One indi- vidual stated: "I have had the opportunity to try anything I considered of value, and 'failure' was as acceptable as 'suc- cess.'" Another person noted: "I would never have taken the chances to attempt these new ways of being if others around me hadn't helped me see the possibilities. Yes—I could do this and this, with their help." Freedom to teach and to ask anyone anything were also mentioned by faculty.

Within this environment, living the philosophy was viewed as both an opportunity and a responsibility. One individual expressed the importance of values in her work:

> Communication, openness, flexibility are the values and actions that are important to me in "living out" and co-creating a work environment. Listening, silence, and prayer are the other side of the soul that I practice.

The responsibility to live out the program philosophy was expressed by another faculty person:

> I believe that the responsibility of living nursing as an expression of being and becoming through caring is an understatement. Not only is it a responsibility, but also a consistent expression of being human, nurse, teacher, practitioner, and person.

Growth, another predominant theme described by faculty, was often linked to unexpected accomplishments. One faculty member reflected this theme in her description of the meaning of group membership:

> So many words come to mind: challenge, hope, exciting, changing, nourishing, fulfilling, exasperating. I would not choose to be a member of any other faculty. In the five years that I have been a member of this group, my own personal growth has been tremendous and I have accomplished more than I ever expected.

Being challenged to grow was a common expression. A professional staff person noted: "I am often asked to do things that I never thought of doing before; writing a chapter in a book, organizing the self-study supporting data, organizing a major conference." Challenge was further expressed by another individual:

> This group provides a challenge for my thoughts and perceptions. At times it is only simple words. At other times it is dialogue. I feel as though my brain is continually stimulated, alive, working, and processing. This should not be taken negatively or appear tiring, as I have never felt so awakened to my inner self. I would say that if I had to summarize the meaning of being a member of this group, I would say "Growth" and "Love."

As the above statement reflects, freedom to grow was consistently linked with encouragement and support from other members of the faculty/professional staff group. This was further described by a professional staff person:

> My experience here at FAU has widened my horizons greatly. I came into this school with a rather narrow, rigid framework and have expanded it greatly. I've learned because of dialogues, reading, discussions, work experiences with students, faculty, other staff; with the Dean, university committees, and class assignments; and in being friends with some of the faculty and staff.
> Like anywhere else, it isn't perfect, but the environment here is much more supportive, open, and friendly than in any other place I've worked in a very long time. I am encouraged to grow—expand—whatever you want to call it, and that is important to me.

Growth was paradoxically described as both a turning inward and an opening outward toward an uncertain future. Turning inward was likened to "returning to my roots in nursing, having traveled far away from them in the 10 years before coming to FAU." This staff person explained:

> By learning the caring philosophy, I began to see how nursing could be exciting for me again, taking me to the place I've really always loved—the person-to-person relationship of nurse and client. Finding out that everything else was on the periphery to this core of nursing helped me make the decision to return to school . . . so that I could broaden my horizons, not only in my nursing life, but in my entire life.

Also reflected in faculty members' comments were the uncertainties of the outcomes of growth. One individual likened this uncertainty to "growing and developing as a colleague toward a new way of being in a university structure." As another faculty person noted, "One never knows quite where one will end up."

SUMMARY

The philosophy contains both constraints and freedoms. Loss of the minority view was expressed as a struggle. Molding to fit the dominant view led to a sense of connectedness. Individuals living within the faculty circle sought both to maintain their own views and to recognize and support the needs of the group. From this struggle, feelings of freedom and growth emerged, as well as respect and support for others. Nevertheless, at the point in time captured by this study, respect for individuals was easier to achieve than respect for the diversity of ideas. In truth, these cannot be separated, and so the struggle to understand and live the philosophy is an ongoing process.

The Experience of Being a Student in a Caring-Based Program

Anita Beckerman, Anne Boykin,
Susan Folden, and Jill Winland-Brown

This chapter focuses on our students. The students are at the heart of our program. They give validity to our efforts. Our caring-based program is "lived" to the extent that we as faculty live it and they as students experience it. It is our belief that faculty in all programs of nursing are committed to relationships with students that reveal respect of person. This chapter, therefore, will not focus on these relationships but on how students come to know self as caring person and the meaning of this knowledge to their practice.

The knowing and living of caring must be transmitted in the fabric of our being. Faculty, however, do not perceive themselves as experts on knowing caring, but as persons continually open to knowing self and other as caring. There is a humility expressed in the desire to continually grow in caring. Caring is not something to be attained but a process of daily becoming. Faculty, with students, continue in this journey of co-discovery. Throughout the program of study, particular value is placed on coming to know students as caring persons. We, as faculty, realize we should create occasions (informal gatherings, daily encounters) whereby faculty and students can come to know each other. This process explicitly speaks to the value of "other" and assists students in understanding the concept of professionhood. It is the belief of the faculty that this focus is essential if nursing is to be lived to its fullest.

WHO ARE THE STUDENTS?

Many generic students have prior degrees and are seeking a second bachelor's degree. The disciplines of students' first degrees include economics, education, medical technology, and humanities, as well as other areas. We have students with master's degrees as well as doctorally prepared persons seeking nursing degrees. The generic baccalaureate students attend school on a full-time basis, but most of them carry multiple responsibilities related to work and families. The average age is 28. Sixty students are admitted annually; of these, 13 percent are male and 15 percent represent minorities.

Our registered nurse students have graduated from local community colleges and are furthering their education (part-time) while continuing to work (full-time). Their average age is 32.

The majority of the students in the master's program in nursing carry a part-time load (one to two courses) while working primarily in managerial positions in a range of nursing practice settings. To date, over 100 students are currently enrolled in the graduate program. Thirty-seven students are at the thesis stage and 20 have graduated.

STUDENT AS CARING PERSON

In keeping with the philosophy, each person is viewed as caring and is free to choose values, aspirations, and desires that give meaning to living. Each person brings unique contributions to the dance of nursing, which was described in Chapter 2. When students enter the program, they are encouraged to better know who they are as person and to authentically live out their uniqueness. This opportunity presents challenges for both faculty and students. Faculty must be open to experiencing and understanding differences, and students must be supported to take the risks necessary to know and to express themselves.

Various strategies are used to facilitate this knowing of self as caring person. Faculty have found the use of guided imagery tapes and other centering exercises helpful. (Not only does this provide students with a framework for coming to know self as person but it also serves as a useful tool for centering as student of professional nursing prior to engaging in each nursing practice situation.) Initially, these experiences are planned by the faculty for the student. These exercises provide students with opportunities to learn how to reach the core of their being; to reflect on their beauty, their uniqueness, and their artistry. The intention, however, is for students to become comfortable with engaging in this exercise at any moment. Student input indicates the value of this approach in coming to know self. Although the particulars of how the knowing occurs are unclear, the reality of its happening has been made explicit.

Students may also choose to enroll in an elective course, Modes of Helping III, in which they study some of the nontraditional ways of healing, such as use of relaxation, music, poetry, and therapeutic touch. It is not expected that students will decide to integrate all these strategies into their own personal lives. However, they may begin to understand that these healing methods are of importance to others and may become of value for them. A few comments from students may illustrate this understanding: "Through this course I learned to relax, rejuvenate, and assess a situation from a different perspective"; "I learned to care for myself so I can care more for patients"; "I have been allowed to learn and to integrate so many new things by observing, participating, and making decisions about them myself."

One strategy that is constant (because of the curriculum structure) is that, in the study of nursing situations, students continually focus on who they are as caring person in a particular nursing situation and how their response to calls for nursing reflects and celebrates the unique gifts they bring to nursing. Through the study of nursing, students learn to conceptualize, think critically, value person as important in itself, and ground decisions and actions in caring. Students are respected as important in themselves, are encouraged to risk discovering their creative selves, and are freed up to promote their being and becoming. Competence and confidence in caring grow through experience.

We offer the following stories, shared by undergraduate generic and registered nurse students as well as by graduate students who were asked about the experience of coming to know self as caring person:

> I grew in unpredictable ways through the study of nursing. Course focus, dialogue and objectives, assigned readings, and clinical and classroom assignments reflect, in depth, the philosophy of "nursing as the process of being and becoming through caring." As a student, I was therefore required to call to consciousness all ways of knowing in order to perceive, understand, and articulate caring in nursing—of environment, self, and others. It is within this exploratory process that I evolved and came to know myself as caring person.

> ———

> Unlike my prior education endeavors, the "world" of nursing is not simply defined by a series of facts and figures created by others for the student to learn and memorize. This world, in addition, possesses a dimension of "depth" which consists of those understandings, feelings, thoughts, and emotions that can only come from within each of us. . . . only through an understanding of these facets that make up the substance of our ability to care do we become able to extend ourselves out to another human being. My nursing education has served me well in promoting this understanding within me and has allowed me to grow in terms of my humanity by allowing to flourish within me that which I long suspected was hidden deep within—the ability to care for another.

> ———

> I feel that I'm perched upon a lily pad in this vast sea of life. . . . My trip to the lily pad was not without struggle. . . . My confidence increased when I realized that each lily pad was unique in its own . . . . How could I

have not noticed all the wonderment around me . . . ?
My consciousness is now expanding more. I'm more
open and sensitive. I take more time to see things deeper
and broader.

———

Through my aesthetic expressions of nursing situations,
I have been able to share very intimate moments of
laughter, sadness, humility, despair, and hope with each
other and come to value each other on a higher level.
This valuing will cultivate caring collegiality in the professional practice of nursing.

———

This program helped me to know self as caring person
by celebrating my personhood, Charlotte as Charlotte.
I have come to know myself more here through a
process of studying and learning in an atmosphere of
celebration of every person's contribution to the community and the anticipation of that person's unfolding
in its own way. I have been a caring person without
knowing the philosophical basis for it and am still trying to fit myself into the concept. I would have to say I
am still in process of coming to know myself as caring
person as a reflection of every person's being in the
world. I have been challenged over the last 5 years to
think and be and have learned so much more of caring
by being cared for.

———

I struggled to grow as nurse, person, and scholar, and
create meaning and order [in] my life as nurse. I im-
mersed myself in the college's philosophy of nursing and
embraced the notion of caring as unique in nursing. Caring connections between student and faculty enlight-
ened my personal knowing of nursing and exposed me
to possibilities in nursing as I was invited and encouraged to view nursing through a new lens, listen for calls

for nursing, and consider my own creative responses to those calls. I discovered that caring in nursing is central to my being as nurse and person, and that all nursing flows from the connectedness I experience with others in need. This discovery freed me to live caring in my day-to-day encounters with patients, families, and colleagues. I felt respected as a person and valued as a human being worthy of kindness and consideration, and enjoyed spiritual growth as I dared to tell my nursing stories and risked sharing myself with others.

———

The concept of devoting an entire curriculum of nursing to caring seemed a redundant and superfluous one; all of us were nurses, and we all *knew* that we were caring, yet not one of us was able to explicitly bring forward how we as nurses expressed our caring for our patients other than through our behavior. We were constantly challenged to examine our beliefs, to learn our prejudices, to stand up for those in our charge. We were taught to love the trust, and to seek truth wherever the road would lead. We learned that nursing is a profession and a discipline that is part of the very essence of what it is to be human, and that the love of the truth engendered in this graduate school will assure that our lives as nurses will be devoted to seeking truth for ourselves as well as for our patients.

These are but a few stories of students, expressing how they came to know self as caring person. From such experiences, which our students in their humility share with us, we have come to believe that a program of study with caring at its core can become real among those wishing to embrace it. As a result of these experiences, students testify repeatedly that knowing self as caring person changes their way of being in the world.

STUDENT AS CARING PROFESSIONAL

Students come to know themselves as unique, special, caring persons who create and live the meaning of their lives. As they begin to know self as caring and cared for, they deepen their knowing of others as caring and worthy of care. Students continue to grow in their understanding of the program's articulated focus of nursing (promoting the process of being and becoming through caring). The courage they found to know self is translated to knowing other in nursing situations. There is a realization of the importance of knowing who the other *is* as well as his or her hopes and dreams for growing through caring.

The following nursing situations were shared by some students as they came to know themselves as caring professionals. An excerpt from a student's journal illustrates the role Carper's patterns of knowing play in helping to articulate nursing as promoting the process of being and becoming through caring.

> This week I nominated a staff nurse for our nursing excellence award for the quarter. As I reflected on which of the nurses would best deserve this award, one particular nurse came to mind. She is one of the kindest nurses I know . . . and has a unique ability to improve health through caring. I now appreciate C. for her special skills as she exemplifies this award for nursing excellence. This is directly related to my learning through this course. When I wrote the summary for the hospital newsletter, describing the nurse receiving the award, I tried something new, writing the piece using the patterns of knowing. Following are excerpts: "C.'s empirical

nursing skills are very well-developed, as are [those of] most Critical Care Nurses. However, C. brings to Nursing an esthetic sense of knowing. She listens to her patients and hears what they are saying. She regularly takes the more critical patients in the ICU . . . . She consistently includes the family in all health care matters and offers support and reassurance. . . . As her Manager, I have been frequently concerned that C. was becoming too emotionally involved with her patients and their families. I have seen her crying with the family and patients (her personal knowing). When it becomes evident to C. that her patients will not survive, she does everything she can to assist the family and the patient to accept the inevitable. Her ethical sense of knowing allows C. to recognize when it is important to allow a patient to die. . . . I have since changed my mind about C.'s involvement with her patients and recognize this now to be her special gift she brings to Nursing. C. *is* what Nursing *is.*"

———

Through the course of the semester and in conjunction with actual nursing practice experience, I learned that there is no one "correct" approach to being in a nursing situation as caring person since caring is co-created in a unique interplay between the nurse and the client (patient) as caring person. My application of caring philosophy and coming to know myself as caring person is best expressed in the following:

BEING THERE

We look at life through the same eyes
And share a bond of understanding.
I want to be sensitive to your needs
Even when words cannot make them known.

Changes are sometimes very painful to bear.
I sense that you feel that you are alone
And that no one could feel how you feel inside.
I know how much you hurt inside
As if somehow the light of happiness
Refuses to shine on you.
I wish that somehow
I could be your light,
But all I can tell you is that sometimes
I hurt too
And all I can do
Is give you
My hand to hold,
My ears to listen,
And my heart
So that I may care
As much for you
As for myself.
Let us come together
So that I may know you completely
And explore the world of possibilities
Of a place free from sadness and pain—
A place far from here.
But if we should fail in our quest,
Let our caring serve to
Buoy us up from our despair.
I can't promise you that
Our quest will be fulfilled
Or that I can remove that
Which shrouds the kind of person
Who I know is there.
All I can do is what
I know how to do.
To care for you and
Let you know
That I am here for you.

And always remember this . . .
That between us
There lives
An unwritten agreement
That says:
    You can count on me.
    You can confide in me.

by Leslie B. Freedman

———

I had cared for the world's most miserable human being, and I dubbed him "the patient from hell." He dwelled on my mind that evening. Why was he the way he was? It really bothered me. I imagined one of my mentors standing before the class asking me, "Who was this man as caring person?" Who was he? Did I really know him or did I really give myself a chance to know him? I realized that I hadn't. At home that night I thought about him a lot in relation to my caring behavior. I recalled part of the college's statement of philosophy of caring, that "the nature of being human is to be caring." I realized that I had to care about him simply because he was a fellow human being. From what I could see going on at the hospital, there was little to show that anyone cared much about him. The next day after classes were over I drove back to the hospital and went to the unit. I found the nurse who was in charge of this patient and asked her how he was doing today. Her eyes rolled back and she let out a big sigh. She needed to say nothing else. I went to his room and knocked on his door. He was trying to eat dinner (without much success). The look on his face was one of puzzlement and surprise when he saw me standing there in my street clothes. I asked him if I could come in and sit with him for a while. "Sure," he curtly replied. His hands were deformed from arthritis and he had trouble holding his utensils. "Unfriendly environment," I thought as I helped him open some of the dinner packaging. I just sat there quietly while he ate. Then he stopped and turned toward me. "Why are you here?", he asked. "I came by to see how you were getting along today," was my reply. "Why?", he shot back. "Because I care about you, I want to help you to take care of yourself." He stopped eating and put down his spoon. Then he told me that I was the first visitor he had since coming to the hospital two weeks earlier. We sat and he began sharing his life with me. What I learned about myself in this instance is representative of my integration of nursing knowledge and personal experience, tempered with a discipline of purposive self-reflection.

———

Several students wrote together: "As ADN graduates pursuing undergraduate degrees in nursing we have been exposed to different nursing curricula. With a caring philosophy, emphasis is placed on the art as well as the science of nursing. The focus of my ADN program was empirical and technological in nature. The philosophy of this program enhanced my nursing practice as therapeutic relationships were enriched through use of all ways of knowing. Nursing education presented within a caring curriculum weaves the fabric of nursing as a whole—the art and the science of nursing."

———

By coming to know myself as caring person I learned to accept myself as I am, value myself as a unique being in this world, and enjoy nursing as a process of caring and connecting with others. I have come to know nursing as a mutually reciprocal process of nurse and client being and becoming through caring. Both the nurse and the one nursed are affected by their interconnectedness, and the spirit of their connectedness lives in stories that represent the nursing situation. Instead of feeling confined or restricted by bureaucracy, I now feel affirmed as a professional nurse free to view nursing situations within bureaucratic structures as possibilities for caring moments and creative responses to calls for nursing. Coming to know self as caring person has afforded this nurse a new lens through which nursing is viewed and the richness of nursing is experienced. Today my practice of nursing is a more gentle, thoughtful practice of creative responses to persons in need. Today I applaud the wonder of nursing and share my knowing of nursing with patients, families, and colleagues. Today nursing is a celebration.

Students are at the heart of our program. We value knowing them as persons and as students of professional nursing. The expressions presented in this chapter confirm that the knowing of self and other as caring person directs their being in nursing practice. It is appropriate to end this chapter with a student's reflection on the courage needed to live out caring in practice:

TO BE OR NOT TO BE

How can I be free to be me?
    I conform, I conform, I conform . . . who might I be?
It is through being with you
    that I learn what I must do.

Caring, caring, caring, is it such a novel concept?
    No, you say, just jump in with both feet.
Why then does the notion haunt me?
    Why do the daily incongruencies taunt me?

I want to participate, to care, to be
    but I keep you separate, separate from me.

Living a Caring-Based Program

I use all the jargon, the intellectual speech
    it keeps me above and you out of reach.

It is through devotion and learning
    that I keep on with my yearning.
For you see, I know I can be me, incongruity-free.
    I have the trust, the faith, they were given to me.

I believe you: to be a caring person
    means to live the meaning of my life.
I have some ideas, that unified aim.
    I have faith that there is nothing but gain.

Dear patients, your eyes are so true,
    there is one promise I give you.
I will to my own self be true.
For then can I care.
    For then can we share
The knowing, the patience, the trust
    will be there.
Freeing me to care.

by Colleen M. Quinn

Researching Experiences of Living Caring

Cheryl Tatano Beck

*I*n this chapter, the characteristics of caring are first explained and exemplified as a basis for discussion of three phenomenological studies. The series of studies was conducted to investigate the meaning of caring throughout a nursing program. The study topics were:

1. The meaning of a caring nursing student–faculty experience.
2. The meaning of caring among nursing students.
3. The meaning of caring experienced among faculty.

All three studies were conducted at Florida Atlantic University's (FAU) College of Nursing.

This chapter then focuses on the common dimensions of caring within a nursing program: authentic presencing, selfless sharing, fortifying support, and uplifting consequences. They have evolved from qualitative research to provide the basis for an emerging middle-range theory of caring. To create a caring environment within a nursing program, these dimensions of caring must be attended to by nurse educators. I suggest specific ways to accomplish this feat.

This chapter is devoted to (1) sharing the hidden aspects of caring that were uncovered in this nursing program and (2) addressing the implications of these findings for nursing educators.

Care is the essence of nursing, as well as the powerful and distinctive attribute of the discipline (Leininger, 1985). Care is becoming a central focus of nursing education. Faculty in schools of nursing are beginning to make care an imperative in teaching, research, and practice (Leininger & Watson, 1990).

An essential challenge of nursing and nursing education is to professionalize human caring through the development of the capacity to care (Roach, 1984). Although all persons have the potential to care, this ability is not uniform. Roach (1987) has asserted that a person's own experience in being cared for and expressing caring influences his or her ability to care. Both faculty and nursing students need to assume responsibility for helping to foster each other's capacity to care. An initial step in developing nursing students' and faculty's ability to care is to surround them with a caring environment. Students and faculty need to have a sense of being cared for if they are to nurture their own ability to care for others.

The capacity to care is not an automatic way of relating to people. Caring responsivity remains dormant if it is not affirmed and actualized (Roach, 1984). The professionalization of human caring in nursing must encompass the significance of caring as responsivity. Caring is a response to value—value in oneself, in the persons who receive the nursing, and in the persons with whom one lives or relates professionally. One of the key motivating factors in persons who choose nursing as a career is their desire to care. Roach has raised the question: Are educational programs designed to capitalize on this source of motivation? An environment where caring models are visible is crucial in the process of nurturing the capacity to care. Care role models are important for learning and for visible care images (Leininger, 1986). Leininger has warned that, without explicit teaching and practice opportunities of care in nursing schools, faculty cannot ensure that their graduates will practice caring later. Leininger has identified nursing faculty as students' key role models of caring. Beck (1992a) has called for nursing students to be care role models for each other. If caring is to permeate a nursing program and spill over to patient care, faculty need to be caring role models not only for their students but also for faculty colleagues. Nursing students need to be care role models not only for their fellow students but also for faculty.

To assist in the discovery and practice of care, Leininger (1986) encouraged the identification of factors that can facilitate caring. She called for the use of qualitative research methods to uncover the covert and embedded aspects of care. Through the examination of nursing students' and faculty members' caring experiences with each other, the meanings assigned to these caring experiences will be better understood by both nursing students and faculty. Care can be facilitated by the sharing of caring experiences with each other. By means of this sharing, a caring ethos can develop in a nursing program, and care can be advanced through these insights (Leininger, 1986).

NURSING STUDENT–FACULTY CARING

In this first study, 47 nursing students were asked to describe in detail a caring experience they had had with a faculty member in the nursing program (Beck, 1991). These written descriptions were analyzed using Colaizzi's (1978) phenomenological method.

From each written description, phrases or sentences that directly pertained to caring between nursing students and faculty were extracted. The meaning of each of these significant statements was spelled out. Next, the formulated meanings from all 47 written descriptions were organized into clusters of themes. An exhaustive description of a caring nursing student–faculty experience was developed from the results of the data analysis and was then validated with the nursing students to ensure that the essence of their caring experience was captured.

Three clusters of themes evolved from this data analysis: (1) attentive presence, (2) sharing of selves, and (3) consequences. By integrating these three theme clusters and their corresponding formulated meanings, the following exhaustive description of a nursing student–faculty member caring experience was developed:

> A faculty member's time is perceived as a valuable gift that is given to a student. In a caring interaction, the student perceives the faculty member as providing an unhurried atmosphere wherein the student does not feel rushed. Through gestures such as smiling, eye contact, touching, and the sharing of a faculty member's own experiences, the student is put at ease. The faculty member

senses something is bothering the student even before the student tells him or her. As a result of the faculty member's attentive listening and undivided attention, the student feels important and valued as a unique person. Respect for the student is evident. A faculty member has a way of making a student feel like a peer. The faculty member makes the student's concerns his or her concerns by putting himself or herself in the student's shoes. Expression of the student's feelings is allowed without the fear of the faculty member being judgmental. Encouragement is given to the student to become motivated to achieve his or her educational goals. The faculty member recognizes a student's accomplishment beyond what the student believes he or she has achieved. Patient, supportive, understanding, and empathetic are additional qualities of a caring faculty member. Voluntarily making the extra effort to follow through on a student's progress with his or her problem impresses the students. A caring interaction not only has a long-lasting effect on a student, but also is contagious. (Beck, 1991, p. 21)

FIVE C'S OF CARING

Caring behaviors of nursing faculty, as identified by nursing students, illustrate the five characteristics of caring put forth by Roach (1984): (1) competence, (2) confidence, (3) compassion, (4) conscience, and (5) commitment.

Competence involves a person's having the knowledge and skills necessary to respond appropriately to the demands of his or her profession and responsibilities. Nursing students repeatedly comment on how the faculty share their knowledge and expertise. The following two excerpts, written by students, describe this sharing of faculty members' knowledge and expertise:

> It was my first clinical experience last fall and it happened to be in the postpartum setting. Not only was I anxious regarding my new skills but I was very anxious regarding handling newborn infants. My instructor emphasized that if we felt unsure about our ability to perform a certain procedure, we should let her know and she would be right there to guide us. My instructor asked if I wished to spend extra time with the infants so as to feel more comfortable. She took me down to the nursery and stayed right there by me while I held the babies and even fed one. She shared tips on how to hold and feed the babies. This greatly alleviated my anxiety. I felt if it weren't for my instructor's receptive, caring attitude and her clinical help at this time, my clinical experience would have been one that I faced daily with dread. Instead, her competence and confidence in this clinical situation made me feel more secure in my skills, less anxious and more positive about the entire clinical experience.

> ———

> Last year we had a pathophysiology clinical situation paper due which was 20 percent of the grade. As I began to look for information, I found it was difficult to find organized material on the ailment assigned to me. After many visits to the library, I found myself in the nursing lab going through books there. A faculty member approached me and inquired what I was up to. I told her and she immediately began to list to me a number of resources and ideas that I could use. She even began to help me look through the books in the lab. I told her I appreciated her help, but that she didn't need to take up

any more of her time paging through books. She said, "No problem, I'd love to help you in any way I can, whenever you need it."

Confidence is the attribute that fosters trusting relationships. Mutual trust and respect are critical aspects of confidence. In the two nursing students' stories that follow, this trust is beautifully addressed:

> I had an appointment to discuss an assignment with my instructor. This turned out to be almost a 1½-hour conversation. We discovered we had many interests in common. When I brought up the subject of the assignment, we got into some very personal observations. The subject was the death of people that were close to us and she allowed me to expose some things I had felt but never talked about before. At the same time, she shared her own experiences. There was a development of trust and understanding.

> ⸻

> During this semester I was undergoing some rough self-evaluation resulting from a problem I had at work. I indirectly hinted at this during one of my journal entries. The faculty member zeroed in on my plea for help and offered guidance and assistance. She set up a meeting with me and during our meeting an interaction of trust, patience, and learning persisted. As I reflect on this moment of sharing, I can truly appreciate and am indebted to her for her concern and the trust she conveyed.

Compassion permits one person to participate in the experience of another, to be sensitive to the pain of another. Compassion involves sharing in another's joys, sorrows, pain, and accomplishments. Excerpts from the nursing students' written accounts continually illustrate the compassion of the faculty: "She shared in my joy and excitement"; "She became attuned to my despairs, especially as I was hurting on the inside"; and "I felt like I was on top of the earth and she shared this feeling with me at the time."

Conscience, the fourth attribute of caring, is a state of moral awareness. Conscience grows out of a process of valuing self and others. Students shared how caring faculty valued them as individuals: "She constantly reinforces my value as a person, a contributing member of society." The following two segments from students' written descriptions of a caring interaction also illustrate faculty's valuing them as individuals:

> I returned to the university on a whim and after one hour's prodding by a friend I decided to take a "bridge" course for the nursing degree. I had all but given up on nursing, was frustrated that I could not maintain enthusiasm for finishing a bachelor's degree. A BSN seemed far too elusive and removed from me. I felt totally inadequate to even consider a BSN degree. The faculty member's caring behavior was gentle acceptance of me—as I presented myself—and a feeling that I had value—worth—and had/have a lot to contribute to the nursing profession and humanity.

> This was a chance encounter in the nursing office after I had taken a challenge exam in pathophysiology the day before I was scheduled for major surgery. I was in the office to take care of another matter when this particular faculty member walked through. She immediately smiled as she always did. She asked what I was up to. I explained I had taken the test as soon as possible because of the approaching surgery and she volunteered to

get the results for me as soon as possible and mail them to me. She personally went downstairs three floors to check on it at that time and came back with the results immediately. This may be a small matter to others but her "caring" showed up in many ways in this situation. She gave of her valuable time. In this world where many times we are just numbers, it is very uplifting to be seen important as an individual.

Commitment, the final C, is the convergence of one person's desires and obligations, what one wants to do and what one is supposed to do. Commitment requires investment of oneself in a task, a person, or a career. "Committed" was an adjective frequently used by the nursing students to describe caring faculty members. For example:

Last fall when I was beginning the clinical phase of the nursing program, I was also dealing with problems at home, namely money and my husband and his two children. I was extremely overwhelmed and decided to talk with a faculty member about formally withdrawing. The professor, without pushing me one way or another, stressed the importance of caring for self. She related her own present and past situations to me and encouraged me to seek out alternative methods of self-help and guidance should I deem them necessary. I remember thinking to myself, "Here is a woman who is so committed, who has so many roles and responsibilities, so many people hold her in high esteem. Yet she's human and she has family problems too, although you'd never know it by looking at her!" The fact that she was so committed to nursing, that she was going on with her life in spite of pressures and problems really stressed the importance of having the courage of your own convictions and standing up for what you really want and need.

CARING AMONG NURSING STUDENTS

The second in this series of phenomenological studies focused on caring among nursing students (Beck, 1992a). In this study, 53 nursing students described, in writing, a situation in which they had experienced caring from another nursing student. Van Kaam's (1966) phenomenological method was used to analyze these written descriptions. First, descriptive expressions of caring among nursing students were identified and categorized into four constituents: (1) authentic presencing, (2) selfless sharing, (3) fortifying support, and (4) enriching effects. Each category or constituent was ranked according to the percentage score derived from the number of times these descriptive expressions were listed by the participants. Next, a hypothetical description of caring among nursing students was written and tested among a random selection of 20 percent of the sample. The description's tryout was successful, and these constituents were synthesized into one description of the total experience of caring among nursing students.

Table 7–1
Constituents of a Caring Experience among Nursing Students, with Sample of 53 Students Expressing Each Constituent

Constituents of Caring	Students Expressing Constituents	
	Number	Percentage
Selfless sharing	50	94%
Enriching effects	47	89
Fortifying support	45	85
Authentic presencing	42	79

The numbers and percentages of the 53 participants expressing each of the four necessary constituents can be found in Table 7–1.

The synthesized description containing these four necessary constituents is given below. Each constituent is followed by a justification and explanation.

The experience of caring between nursing students occurs under an umbrella of authentic presencing where selfless sharing and fortifying support lead to enriching effects.

Authentic presencing.
Nursing students can sense when a fellow student needs caring even before that student says anything. Listening is a major component of authentic presencing.

Selfless sharing.
A caring nursing student gives of himself/herself unselfishly, without expectations of receiving anything in return. He or she shares knowledge, expertise, experiences, thoughts, feelings, and time with another nursing student. In a nursing student's hectic life, where time is a valued commodity, the sharing of this time with a fellow nursing student is perceived as a precious gift. Most often, this sharing is unsolicited.

Fortifying support.
Encouragement and unquestioning assistance are given to a nursing student who many times is only an acquaintance.

Enriching effects.
A caring experience with another nursing student has both immediate and long-term outcomes. Immediately after the caring experience, a nursing student feels good that someone was thinking of him or her. Gratitude toward the caring nursing student frequently was

expressed. Long-term consequences included aspects of learning caring and its contagious nature. By experiencing a caring experience, nursing students revealed that they, in turn, learned how to care for others. Caring is contagious. Once a nursing student experienced caring, he or she wanted to care for other nursing students in the same manner.

The following extracts from students' written descriptions of caring experiences between nursing students illustrate the four necessary constituents:

Authentic presencing, selfless sharing, and fortifying support.
It was a tough semester. Lots of demands on time. Pulled in all different ways . . . home, school, work. It would have been so easy to quit. All I needed was something else to go wrong. A fellow nursing student sensed this, recognized it, and didn't criticize me but really listened to my complaints, spent extra time going over work I found hard, and encouraged me to stay with it—not by any real overt action but mostly by giving support.

Selfless sharing.
A fellow nursing student, who was aware of how tight my time schedule was, copied reserve articles for me on a weekly basis throughout my entire statistics course. To me this meant a great deal. She was willing to sacrifice an hour she could have been relaxing but she made the effort so my life would be easier. Since we both worked full-time and were carrying 15 hours that semester, she knew that time was a premium commodity.

Selfless sharing and enriching effects.
In lab, we were to decipher instructions from a kardex, go to the medication cart, and remove the correct dosage. I had not prepared for this class enough and did not understand some of the abbreviations. A fellow

nursing student shared her knowledge and helped me understand my patient's card. I never asked for her help. She just volunteered it. I am usually a very good student and I have a low opinion of others who do not commit the time and energy to studying that I do. Her act of caring made me feel ashamed and guilty for not extending her unjudgmental caring to others. I hope I can care for another nursing student in the future the way she cared for me.

Fortifying support and enriching effects.
I attended the afternoon statistics class the following week after our first exam. The next day I received a phone call from another nursing student who was very concerned that I had withdrawn from class due to the exam. She was prepared to discuss all the reasons why I should stay in the class and offered her support to help me through the statistics course. For one moment I realized that someone who I only know from class really cared for me. This made me feel good about myself. It encouraged me to move on, knowing I was not in this alone. I was able to care for this and other nursing students in a more open way because of this caring experience.

CARING EXPERIENCES AMONG FACULTY

In this third study, 17 nursing faculty participated in exploring the meaning of caring as experienced among faculty. Faculty were asked to describe in detail a caring experience they had had with another nursing faculty member. Van Kaam's (1966) phenomenological method was used to analyze these written caring descriptions.

Four necessary constituents of a caring experience among faculty emerged: (1) authentic presencing, (2) unconditional support, (3) spontaneous sharing, and (4) uplifting consequences. The numbers and percentages of the 17 participants expressing each of these four necessary constituents are presented in Table 7–2.

The constituents were synthesized into one description, to identify the total caring experience among nursing faculty. The synthesized description containing these four necessary constituents is given below. Each constituent is followed by a justification and explanation.

> The experience of caring between nursing faculty is encompassed in authentic presencing and abounds with unconditional support and spontaneous sharing from which emanate uplifting consequences.

Authentic presencing.
Words are not needed between nursing faculty to convey the need for caring. Faculty can sense when a fellow faculty member needs caring even before that faculty member speaks of this desire. A caring faculty member is

Table 7–2
Constituents of a Caring Experience among Nursing Faculty, with Sample of 17 Faculty Expressing Each Constituent

	Faculty Expressing Constituents	
Constituents of Caring	Number	Percentage
Unconditional support	15	88%
Spontaneous sharing	15	88
Uplifting consequences	15	88
Authentic presencing	11	65

truly there for his or her colleague. Active listening, while blocking out all other concerns, is an integral ingredient in authentic presencing.

Unconditional support.
The sustaining encouragement and support of caring faculty was not asked for but was voluntarily, eagerly, and freely given. It was not necessary for faculty to have known each other for any extended period of time before this support occurred. Caring faculty never asked or expected anything in return for this support, not even recognition.

Spontaneous sharing.
Caring faculty took the initiative to share themselves with their fellow faculty members. This sharing consisted of voluntarily offering and giving of faculty's valuable time, which was a limited commodity. A sharing of ideas, course materials, opposing views, hugs, expertise, etc., was exchanged.

Uplifting consequences.
As a result of another faculty member's caring, faculty felt valued and respected as person. Through this nurturing, caring was contagious. Faculty who had experienced this caring desired, in turn, to care for another faculty member.

The following quotes from faculty's written descriptions of caring between faculty illustrate the four necessary constituents:

Authentic presencing.
While we were getting coffee, she sensed something was bothering me. Even though she had a tight schedule that morning, she took the time and sat right down with me and asked if there was anything she could do for me.

While I explained to her what was wrong, she listened intensely and gave her total attention to me.

Unconditional support.

I have never felt that kind of support from peers before. They were all there from the beginning through to the end. Their faith and trust in me was wonderful. I don't believe I will ever be able to thank all of them. When you feel this sincere type of support, just their presence is enough to make you feel a part of something much greater than just a group of faculty.

Spontaneous sharing.

When I was newly hired, a faculty member shared with me all of her course materials because I would be teaching her class. This may sound like nothing but the open generosity was remarkable. She did not know me. Not only did she share course work but she shared the meaning of being a faculty member in nursing at FAU. I felt that she definitely went out of her way to someone she had never met before.

Uplifting consequences.

I felt like I was really known and valued. It was not that I wasn't sure of that already, but her making the effort to tell me brought it home to me in the concrete present, and I felt truly cared for. The experience made me more aware, more committed. It encouraged me to make the effort with others. I think it has something to do with making the effort to extend oneself in a personal way.

Valuing and practicing these four necessary constituents of caring among nursing faculty will affirm and actualize faculty's capacity to care. Once fortified from being cared for, faculty members will, in turn, be better able to nurture their own ability to care for others, be they students, other faculty, or patients.

DIMENSIONS OF CARING
WITHIN A NURSING PROGRAM

After this series of phenomenological research studies was completed, four dimensions of caring within a nursing program were identified as being common to all three studies: (1) authentic presencing, (2) selfless sharing, (3) fortifying support, and (4) uplifting consequences. These dimensions provided the beginning work on an emerging middle-range theory of caring. Through this qualitative research on the meaning of caring for both faculty and nursing students, the essential components of caring within a nursing program were uncovered. Promoting these four dimensions of caring can help to create, within a nursing program, a caring environment where faculty's and students' capacity to care can be nurtured and caring can flourish.

The four dimensions of caring that permeated all three studies emerged from the constituents determined in each of the research studies (see Table 7–3).

Authentic Presencing

Authentic presencing is a striving to enter the world of the other—the world of a nursing faculty member or a nursing student. Attentive listening is essential if authentic presencing is to occur. By focusing one's complete attention on the nursing student or faculty member, one conveys to that person that he or she is truly heard and understood. The faculty member or student who is caring can sense that something is bothering another person. The need for caring is known even before that person verbalizes it.

Table 7–3
Origins, within Research Studies, of the Four
Necessary Constituents of an Emerging Theory of
Caring within a Nursing Program

Study I: Caring between Nursing Students and Faculty	Study II: Caring between Nursing Students	Study III: Caring between Faculty
Attentive presence	Authentic presencing	Authentic presencing
Sharing of selves	Selfless sharing	Spontaneous sharing
Consequences	Enriching effects	Uplifting consequences
Support	Fortifying support	Unconditional support

The following quotes from the first study on caring (between faculty and nursing students) illustrate authentic presencing:

> I get goose pimples every time I think of this beautiful experience although it happened over 2 years ago. Thank God she did not trivialize this episode but, rather, listened as all nurses should listen, not to the words or what happened, but to the part that is pouring from the heart. And because she did that, I am happy, healthy, productive, and a worthwhile human being today.

> ———

> The most significant thing that I remember from her was that she stopped what she was doing and listened to me. She gave me her full attention. She acknowledged the loss I must be feeling and did not minimize the situation. She communicated that she cared through her eye contact, expression, touching, and total attention.

Selfless Sharing

Sharing involves unselfishly and spontaneously giving of one-self without expectation of receiving anything in return. The giving of faculty members' and students' time is viewed as a precious gift. Knowledge, expertise, experiences, ideas, feelings, and self are all shared.

The following excerpts from nursing students' written caring descriptions illustrate the theme of sharing and its importance within a nursing program where one's time is such a valued commodity:

> Back in March of last semester I had a severe personal tragedy in my life. I called a friend of mine (fellow student) and told her how distraught I was. She came right over, helped me to get myself together. It wasn't that she eased much of the pain I was in that was important, since the magnitude of my problem was so intense, that I still am suffering from some of the aftershock. The importance was that she was there, was there quickly, and gave of her valuable time without questioning me, fully knowing that there was no reward to be reaped. This was caring.

———

> I was having a difficult time in one of my classes—and at midterm I still had no idea what the instructor was talking about. This particular student spent about an hour with me over the phone and in several meetings during breaks of the class. She had had much of this information in a previous class and was well-versed in the language of this particular theory and its abstract ideas. It made me feel good inside to know she would help me when I was struggling. My anxiety was relieved immediately. I felt like she cared enough to take the time and

teach me the language and basic concepts. I felt better going into midterms and finals. I felt better at the class. I didn't feel so "stupid" now. She was very patient and kind, very knowledgeable.

Fortifying Support

The third dimension of caring within a nursing program, support, is unconditional and fortifying. This support is unsolicited and freely given without anything expected in return. Sustaining encouragement frequently provides a pillar on which to lean. Knowing a student or faculty member for any extended period of time is definitely not a prerequisite for providing support.

The following passage from a faculty member's description of caring she had received from another faculty member exemplifies this dimension of support:

> I worked very closely with this faculty member during the organization of the self-study report. I had never been through that experience before and wasn't sure what I was doing. I was so anxious about it at first that I wasn't sure the project could be completed on time. This faculty member was always there for me, to answer my questions, give me guidance as to where I might go for information. I felt valued as a person by her, not just for what I did. I think the work was made a lot easier for me knowing there was one person I could turn to for advice and support, someone who would listen and take the time to talk with me. I knew the support was always there for me, and it made this huge job bearable.

From the study on caring among nursing students has come this excerpt illustrating fortifying support:

I had a beautiful experience with several of my fellow nursing students. I was surprised with an award during a meeting with many of my friends at the school. I was elated at being given the award; however, an even greater reward was the feeling of closeness, respect, caring, and love that they expressed toward me. When I looked over at them, I saw tears streaming down some of their faces. The pride that I saw gleaming from the face of one of my friends is something I will never forget. The support given me was so immense, I felt I could touch it. It became a part of me and a bond even stronger emerged. I grew tenfold as a person that day.

Uplifting Consequences

This fourth dimension of caring has both short- and long-term outcomes. Immediately after a caring experience, nursing faculty and students feel respected and valued as persons and as individuals. As a result of caring, faculty and students feel nurtured. Reminiscing about the caring experience, even years later, energizes and rejuvenates the recipient of this caring. After experiencing a caring interaction, nursing faculty and students have a strong desire to, in turn, reach out to someone else through caring. Caring is contagious. By experiencing caring firsthand, a person learns how to care for others.

Excerpts from all three caring studies repeatedly expressed the uplifting and enriching effects of caring experienced by both nursing faculty and students.

From the nursing student–faculty study have come the following quotes:

I shall never forget that day in her office. It was truly a moment that could have changed my destiny. Because at that moment I made the decision to tough it out and see if I could make it. That was over a year ago. I hope

113

someday I will be able to fully express to this faculty member how much her kindness and caring meant to me.

_____

I pull out the faculty member's letter and get rejuvenated over and over again, reliving the experience. It refreshes the same caring I felt from her.

_____

Anyone could have advised me on what classes to take but it took a very special person to see the fright and insecurity I had hidden within myself. Till this day I don't know how to thank this faculty member. I really don't even know if she realized what she did. But I can honestly say that this individual has been the source of my success today.

From the caring-among-faculty study, the following excerpt illustrates the contagious nature of caring:

A colleague told me that she and several others had been talking about an impending possibility that I would be leaving the faculty at my own initiative. She said that she realized how difficult it would be to replace me. I felt grateful to her for taking the initiative to share her thoughts with me. I felt like I was really known and valued. It was not that I wasn't sure of that already, but her making the effort to tell me brought it home to me in the concrete present, and I felt truly cared for. The experience made me more aware, more committed, [and encouraged me] to make the effort with others.

From the study on caring among nursing students has come a summary quote: "Because of this caring experience, I was able to care for this and other nursing students in a more open way."

Through these three phenomenological studies, the caring dimensions of *authentic presencing, selfless caring, fortifying support,* and *uplifting consequences* were empirically identified and described. By combining the results of the three studies, a definition of caring emerged that captured the essence of caring within a nursing program: *Caring is centered in authentic presencing where selfless sharing and fortifying support flourish and lead to uplifting consequences.*

DISCUSSION

The four dimensions of caring within a nursing program, which have evolved from the three phenomenological studies, constitute the beginnings of an emerging middle-range theory of caring within a nursing program. These dimensions are supported by earlier studies that initiated investigation of caring within a nursing program.

The experience of caring in the teaching–learning process of nursing education was explored by Miller, Haber, and Byrne (1990) in a phenomenological study that confirmed the dimensions of fortifying support and uplifting consequences. In Miller et al.'s study, six senior nursing students described a caring teaching–learning interaction that they had experienced during one of their nursing courses. A caring teaching–learning encounter was described by the students as a process characterized by a pervasive climate of support. This process begins when a perceived need of a student is either anticipated or recognized by a faculty member or when a student brings a concern or problem to a teacher. The faculty member's holistic concern for the student, both personally and academically, is perceived by the student as an essential dimension of the caring encounter. A caring faculty member reaches out to students in an empathetic way, offering a constant presence. Caring interactions as perceived by nursing students involve the mutual and simultaneous dimensions of intimacy, connectedness, trust, sharing, and respect. As a result of these caring interactions, students experienced increased self-worth, self-esteem, and self-confidence.

In Nelms's (1990) phenomenological study of the lived experience of nursing education, 17 generic nursing students were interviewed. A theme that emerged as very meaningful to the lived experiences of these students was their support systems along their educational journey. Their strongest sense of support came from fellow nursing students, and their next strongest, from nursing faculty. The placing of support received from fellow nursing students as number one is reflective of the fortifying support students revealed in the second study described in this chapter (caring among nursing students).

Halldorsdottir (1990) interviewed 9 former nursing students regarding a caring encounter they had had with a faculty member. Phenomenological analysis revealed that a caring encounter with a teacher, from the nursing student's perspective, had four basic components: (1) the teacher's professional caring approach, (2) the resulting mutual trust, (3) a professional teacher–student working relationship, and (4) positive student responses to the caring encounter. Essential components of the teacher's professional caring approach were: professional competence, genuine concern, positive personality, and professional commitment.

The students' positive responses to professional caring very much patterned the dimension of uplifting consequences, which emerged from the series of phenomenological studies conducted on caring within a nursing program. Halldorsdottir (1990) reported four major themes in regard to the positive student responses: (1) sense of acceptance and self-worth, (2) personal and professional growth and motivation, (3) appreciation and role modeling, and (4) long-term gratitude and respect. Students expressed their desire to model themselves on the caring teacher.

Hughes (1992) conducted a qualitative, descriptive study of the student-perceived climate for caring, using a sample of 10 junior nursing students. Data analysis was guided by Noddings' (1984, 1988) components of a moral education: modeling, dialogue, practice, and confirmation. Under the category of modeling, the following subcategories of faculty behaviors were perceived in Hughes's study as caring emerged: (1) displacement of motivation, (2) equality of interaction, (3) presence, (4) prosocial orientation, (5) sensitivity, (6) constancy, (7) personal interest, (8) professional credibility, and (9) ethical responsibility as a teacher. The dominant subcategory was presence: faculty behaviors that conveyed a readiness to make oneself available to a student and to generously invest oneself in another. (Hughes's subcategory of presence confirms the caring constituent of fortifying support in my series of studies.) Nursing students in Hughes's study identified the caring of faculty with an open-door policy: faculty were always there for the students when they needed them. Under the category of dialogue, nursing students described caring as a mutual sharing of faculty and students' thoughts, ideas, and feelings.

The caring constituent of uplifting consequences, particularly the contagious nature of being a recipient of caring, was also supported in Hughes's (1992) study. In the practice category, students revealed their desire to emulate in their future practice those faculty who had enacted caring behaviors.

Swanson (1991) developed a middle-range theory of caring that was inductively derived through three phenomenological studies with disparate sample groups: (1) 20 women who had recently miscarried, (2) 19 care providers in the newborn intensive care unit, and (3) 8 young mothers who had received a long-term public health nursing intervention. The caring processes identified were: knowing, being with, doing for, enabling, and maintaining belief.

Some subdimensions of Swanson's (1991) caring processes are similar to the caring constituents that emerged from my studies on caring within a nursing program. One of the subdimensions of Swanson's caring process of knowing is "centering on the one cared-for." "Being there" is a subdimension of the caring process of being with. Both of these subdimensions fit with my caring constituent of authentic presencing, discussed earlier. "Sharing feelings," another subdimension of Swanson's caring process of being with, touches on a portion of my caring constituent of selfless sharing. Multiple subdimensions of Swanson's caring process of maintaining belief—such as "believing in" and "going the distance"—and her subdimension of "supporting," in the caring process of enabling, speak to my caring constituent of fortifying support.

Three of my constituents of caring—authentic presencing, selfless sharing, and uplifting consequences—are similar to the necessary constituents of nursing students' caring with physically/mentally handicapped children: authentic presencing, reciprocal sharing, and unanticipated self-transformation (Beck, 1992b). In this phenomenological study, Beck explored the meaning of 36 nursing students' caring with exceptional children. The six necessary constituents of caring that emerged from the students' descriptions of their caring experiences were synthesized into the following description: A caring nursing student–exceptional child experience is an interweaving of authentic presencing with physical connectedness and reciprocal sharing overflowing into delightful merriment, bolstered self-esteem, and an unanticipated self-transformation.

In my second study, discussed earlier in the chapter, the selfless sharing that occurred in a caring experience between nursing students differed somewhat from the reciprocal sharing reported with special-needs children. With physically/ mentally handicapped children, reciprocal sharing involved a mutual sharing of selves and of dreams for the future. The selfless sharing that transpired in a caring experience between nursing students was, at times, more one-sided. Caring experiences shared by the nursing students occurred during more of a crisis period for the students; the caring experiences with special-needs children took place during their everyday lives at school.

The unanticipated self-transformation that occurred in nursing students after their caring experiences with exceptional children included unexpected changes in their attitudes toward these special children. Their unforgettable experiences with the physically and mentally handicapped children inspired the nursing students—further support for my caring constituent of uplifting consequences.

IMPLICATIONS FOR NURSE EDUCATORS

Caring is centered in authentic presencing where selfless sharing and fortifying support flourish and lead to uplifting consequences. This definition of caring, which evolved from the three phenomenological studies discussed earlier in the chapter, captures the essence of caring within a nursing program.

To create a caring environment within a nursing program, authentic presencing, selfless sharing, fortifying support, and uplifting consequences must be attended to. Constant vigilance must be kept by both faculty and nursing students if these caring dimensions are to permeate the nursing program. In what specific ways can this feat be accomplished?

If faculty are to help foster nursing students' capacity to care, the first step is to surround the students with a caring environment. To nurture their own ability to care for others, students need to have a sense of being cared for. The empirical findings of the study on the meaning of caring experiences between nursing students and faculty can help nursing educators to know some of the specific behaviors students perceive as caring. With these hidden aspects of caring uncovered, nursing faculty can incorporate these behaviors into their day-to-day encounters with students in both the classroom and clinical arenas. For example, authentic presencing was repeatedly shared by nursing students as a critical ingredient that makes up faculty caring. No matter why a student interacts with faculty, faculty need to give undivided attention to the student. Listening attentively to what the students are saying—or, in some cases, not saying—makes students feel they are being cared for. Not feeling rushed by faculty is highly valued by nursing students as caring. One of the most precious caring gifts faculty can give their students is their time. Faculty need to perfect the art of giving each student the impression that they have all the time in the world for *this* student's concerns.

Being consciously aware of their own nonverbal behavior when talking with students will allow faculty to project the unhurried atmosphere so valued by the students. When students enter a professor's office for a scheduled or unscheduled appointment, faculty should attend to small details—putting down the pen or pencil if they were writing, or sitting down if they were standing. These nonverbal behaviors can convey to students that faculty value them as individuals and are interested in what they have to say.

Nursing students learn caring by experiencing caring practices not only with faculty but also with their fellow nursing students. Use of nursing students as role models of caring is an untapped resource that is readily available in a nursing program. As evidenced by Beck's (1992a) phenomenological study on caring among nursing students, caring can be learned from fellow nursing students. Students who are exemplars of caring for their fellow nursing students need to be valued and rewarded. For example, a bulletin board can be reserved in the school of nursing specifically to highlight exemplars of caring. Students' narratives of caring experiences with faculty, fellow nursing students, or their patients can be posted. Caring can then be visibly valued, promoted, and recognized in nursing education settings.

Before nursing students can understand the individual who needs caring, they have to grow in insight about themselves as caring persons (Bush, 1988). Sharing the four necessary constituents of caring revealed in my studies can help nursing students to begin to examine their own caring actions. Students can be encouraged to reflect on the meaning and experiences of caring. Nurses will be more able to provide care if they know what it is, how it looks in practice, and how it is transacted interpersonally (Roberts, 1990). Caring in nursing students can be facilitated by encouraging them to share their caring experiences and feelings with one another. For example, time in postconferences on the clinical units should be set aside for sharing of "caring moments" that occurred that day. Caring moments can be related to caring experiences with patients, with faculty, or with fellow students.

To create a caring environment throughout a nursing program, not only the nursing students' but also the faculty's capacity to care must be nurtured. Faculty need to rely on each other for caring. Fortifying experiences of being cared for by other faculty can, in turn, help faculty to care for their students. Another source of caring for faculty can be their nursing students. Noddings (1984) believes that the nursing student can be the one who is caring and the educator can be the recipient of caring.

Through experiencing caring, faculty's and students' capacity to care will be nurtured and will grow. Caring responsivity will be affirmed and actualized. One learns caring through interaction with others, wherein one experiences being the recipient of caring, and through opportunities in which a person can see and use the self as caring. Noddings (1984), in her ethic of caring and moral education, reemphasizes that faculty must provide a climate that permits students to internalize caring behaviors.

Seminars and workshops can be held to teach faculty and nursing students the essential elements of caring that have emerged from nursing research studies. Each time a new class of nursing students is admitted, the caring seminars can be repeated. A portion of the orientation of new professors joining the nursing faculty can center on sharing with them the caring materials presented at these seminars.

In a caring-based curriculum, caring needs to be ever present and recognized. Caring should be threaded throughout every course. In nursing research courses, for example, there is a wealth of exciting opportunities to help create and maintain a caring environment. Over the semester, students can be actively involved in a research study on caring. One option is to have nursing students be participants in a caring study conducted by the faculty member teaching the research course. Throughout the semester, the faculty and students can analyze the data and see what findings emerged. Another option is to have the nursing students conduct their own small research projects on caring as one of the class requirements. These caring research projects can be done in small groups.

Weaving research on caring into clinical courses is another exciting method to help create a caring environment throughout a nursing program. For example, at FAU, in one of the three nursing practice courses required for RN to BSN students, the RN students became actively involved in a phenomenological study of a caring nurse–client experience from the perspective of clients experiencing long-term health alterations (Beck, 1993). Each RN student asked one of his or her clients with a chronic health problem: "Please describe a caring experience you have had with a nurse. Write all your thoughts, feelings, and perceptions until you have no more to write." Each week over the semester, a portion of the clinical conferences was devoted to the RN students' analyzing, as a group and with faculty assistance, these written descriptions of caring.

Van Kaam's (1966) phenomenological method was used to obtain the essence of a caring nurse–client experience. The first step in this phenomenological method is to dwell with the data by reading and rereading the written descriptions. As the faculty member read aloud for the first time the clients' descriptions of their caring interactions with nurses, she looked up to see tears in the eyes of her students. Caring was coming alive for these RN students as they entered the world of their clients through the data they had collected. From their weekly data analysis, the following identification and description of the essence of a caring nurse–client experience emerged: "A caring experience between a nurse and a client with a chronic health alteration involves a nurturing engagement by a guardian who provides enlightenment grounded in reliance" (Beck, 1993).

In this course, clinical conferences periodically focused on the RN students' reflecting on their own nursing practice and on whether their practice included any of the caring behaviors identified by the clients in their research. Strategies for incorporating these caring behaviors into their nursing practice were discussed by the RN students.

Roberts (1990) has alerted nurses that they need to uncover more of the characteristics of caring practices so that caring can be recognized, rewarded, and taught. Engaging nursing students and faculty in such caring research studies is one way this can be accomplished within a nursing program. In addition, a caring curriculum can be based on emerging research results.

The varied strategies offered here to create a caring environment will allow caring to be visibly valued, promoted, and recognized in nursing education settings.

REFERENCES

Beck, C. (1993). Integrating research in an RN to BSN clinical course. *Western Journal of Nursing Research, 15*, 118–121.

Beck, C. (1991). How students perceive faculty caring: A phenomenological study. *Nurse Educator, 16*, 18–22.

Beck, C. (1992a). Caring among nursing students. *Nursing Educator, 17*, 22–27.

Beck, C. (1992b). Caring between nursing students and physically/mentally handicapped children: A phenomenological study. *Journal of Nursing Education, 31*, 361–366.

Bush, H. (1988). The caring teacher of nursing. In M. Leininger (Ed.), *Care: Discovery and uses in clinical and community nursing.* Detroit: Wayne State University Press.

Colaizzi, P. (1978). Psychological research as the phenomenologist views it. In R. Valle & M. King (eds.), *Existential–phenomenological alternatives for psychology.* New York: Oxford University Press.

Halldorsdottir, S. (1990). The essential structure of a caring and an uncaring encounter with a teacher: The perspective of the nursing student. In M. Leininger & J. Watson (Eds.), *The caring imperative in education* (pp. 95–108). New York: National League for Nursing.

Hughes, L. (1992). Faculty–student interactions and the student-perceived climate for caring. *Advances in Nursing Science, 14,* 60–71.

Leininger, M. (1985). Transcultural caring diversity and universality: A theory of nursing. *Nursing and Health Care, 6,* 209–212.

Leininger, M. (1986). Care facilitation and resistance factors in the culture of nursing. *Topics in Clinical Nursing, 8,* 1–12.

Leininger, M., & Watson, J. (Eds.). (1990). *The caring imperative in education.* New York: National League for Nursing.

Miller, B., Haber, J., & Byrne, M. (1990). The experience of caring in the teaching–learning process of nursing education: Student and teacher perspectives. In M. Leininger & J. Watson (Eds.), *The caring imperative in education* (pp. 125–135). New York: National League for Nursing.

Nelms, T. (1990). The lived experience in nursing education: A phenomenological study. In M. Leininger & J. Watson (Eds.), *The caring imperative in education* (pp. 285–297). New York: National League for Nursing.

Noddings, N. (1984). *Caring: A feminist approach to ethics and moral education.* Berkeley: University of California Press.

Noddings, N. (1988). An ethic of caring and its implications for instructional arrangements. *American Journal of Education, 96,* 215–230.

Roach, M. S. (1984). *Caring: The human mode of being, implications for nursing.* Toronto: Faculty of Nursing, University of Toronto, Perspectives in Caring Monograph 1.

Roach, M. S. (1987). *The human act of caring: A blueprint for health professions.* Ottawa: Canada Hospital Association.

Roberts, J. (1990). Uncovering hidden caring. *Nursing Outlook, 38,* 67–69.

Swanson, K. (1991). Empirical development of a middle-range theory of caring. *Nursing Research, 40,* 161–166.

Van Kaam, A. (1966). *Existential foundations of psychology.* Pittsburgh: Duquesne University Press.

8

Prizing, Valuing, and Growing in a Caring-Based Program

Savina Schoenhofer and Sherrilyn Coffman

*T*he concept and practice of evaluation within the College of Nursing at Florida Atlantic University (FAU) derive from beliefs about person, nursing, and education, as expressed in the philosophy of the program. Central to the evaluation component is the assumption that the nature of being human is to be caring and to be free to choose values, aspirations, and desires that give meaning to living.

Further, the faculty believes that valid scholarship and practice in nursing require creative integration of knowing and caring. In a caring environment that is supportive for learning, all aspects of the human person are respected, nurtured, and celebrated.

Within this framework, evaluation must be approached as more than objectives, compliance, outcomes, and measurement. The terms *prizing, valuing,* and *growing* describe aims and processes more relevant to our conceptualization of the discipline of nursing than the Tylerian paradigm of educational evaluation. Whether the component being evaluated is administration, students, curriculum, faculty, or resources, it is necessary to live caring values such as honesty, humility, knowing, presence, and connectedness in the evaluation process. In the context of the caring framework, this means that the human freedom to imagine, to hope, to choose, to be in authentic relationship, and to create meaning is what structures those activities traditionally termed *evaluation.*

As with other dimensions of creating a program of nursing education grounded in caring, faculty and students struggle to transcend restricting patterns while actively seeking new and congruent ways of ensuring quality. Each of us comes with a history and with expectations. Faculty come from experiences in programs of nursing education that have valued traditions. Each faculty member who joins a caring-based program must examine traditional patterns in relation to an explicit philosophy of caring. This often leads to a period of experimentation and, at times, to frustration. Most students come with some expectations that are congruent with the caring foundations of nursing but have other expectations that have originated in the impersonality of inflexible institutions. This tension between known ways of being and hopes for new ways of being is felt in the area of evaluation as well as in other aspects of the program.

The FAU faculty has developed a written plan that serves as a strategic guide to evaluation activities within the overall framework of caring. This strategic plan is similar to plans found in many other programs; it includes the categories of subject/content of evaluation, input, general process, timetable, outcome or product of the evaluation strategy, and implementation of decisions following an evaluation. The strategic plan is treated as an adjunct to organization; it contributes to means and is not an end in itself. The strategic plan relies on the underlying philosophy to suggest answers to fundamental questions of why and how. In a caring-based program, formal evaluation processes are recognized as opportunities to grow, rather than being addressed as token compliance or threats to the status quo. Caring concepts such as creativity, responsibility, and unfolding give an important impetus to evaluation.

This chapter addresses evaluation in all the major components of the program: curriculum, students, faculty, administration, and resources.

CURRICULUM

The curriculum, as the shared study of nursing, is the central component with which the other components interrelate. The curriculum represents the embodied beliefs about the nature of the discipline of nursing; these beliefs suggest general characteristics of faculty, students, administration, and resources.

Because curriculum evaluation as an inherent aspect of the shared study of nursing is ongoing, it cannot be viewed separately from faculty and student evaluation. Let's examine a hypothetical though not uncommon example. A member of the faculty, reflecting on a disappointing morning in the classroom, may have the insight that the study of nursing was set aside in favor of a topic from microbiology. That insight may send the faculty person back to the course description and the conceptual framework, in an effort to see whether those documents might be instructive or, perhaps, were lacking as guides. Most likely, the faculty person would share the disappointing experience with a colleague and invite dialogue. To extend the example, a student in the class may similarly experience dissonance and reflect on the relative limits/unfolding possibilities of this particular shared study of nursing. Both the student and the faculty member have access to structures for formalizing their concerns about the curriculum. At the conclusion of every semester, students and faculty are invited to articulate their valuing of courses, their prizing of experiences of shared study, and their suggestions for the unfolding of the curriculum. This input is sought from faculty in response to the following questions:

1. How does each item reflect your current understanding of the philosophy and framework?
   A. Course description
   B. Objectives
   C. Topics
   D. Projects, papers, other assigned activities
2. Is the students' prerequisite knowledge adequate?
   A. Did the students possess a strong knowledge foundation to prepare them for the content of this course? What knowledge could be strengthened?
   B. Were the students able to integrate multiple sources of knowledge necessary for nursing?

3. Recommendations for change based on above analysis:

    A. Specific to the course

    B. In respect to the curriculum as a whole

4. What would you like to say about this course that has not been addressed in the above questions?

Formal student input is sought at the end of each course. In addition to the formal (written) course evaluations, most faculty make it a practice to engage students in dialogue during and at the end of their courses, regarding the students' valuing and prizing of the courses and the growth issues they would recommend. This dialogue evolves as students progress from the first to the final courses in the curriculum and gain experience with the whole. Course evaluation dialogues are viewed as teaching/learning opportunities for both student and faculty; they provide another way to put the entire valuing, prizing, and growing process in the context of caring.

The formal student input obtained at the end of each classroom-based course covers the following points of discussion. Students assign a scaled number to each item and provide written comments:

1. The course content reflected the course objectives.

2. The written assignments and required projects corresponded to the course objectives.

3. Written papers were beneficial for enhancing and supplementing course content to meet the objectives.

4. Exams reflected the course objectives and outcomes.

5. In terms of your personal growth, how would you rate this course?

6. What suggestions do you have for change? (Comment on required texts and readings. Feel free to use additional space.)

Clinical courses are evaluated at the end of each term, using a similar format:

1. Clinical laboratory experiences provided learning to meet course objectives.

2. In terms of your personal and professional growth, how would you rate this course?

3. Which clinical experiences in the course were especially effective in meeting course objectives? Why?

4. Were any clinical experiences not effective in meeting course objectives? Why?

5. What suggestions do you have for change? (Feel free to use additional space.)

The Committee on Curriculum, comprised of faculty members and students from all levels of the program, compiles these evaluations and integrates them into specific curriculum proposals taken to the faculty.

In addition, on a 3-year cycle, the entire curriculum is studied and modifications are worked out. Questions concerning the curriculum might include the following:

- To what extent do curriculum structures demonstrate respect for persons as caring?

- Do teaching/learning activities maximize authentic relating in the classroom? in the direct care setting?

- Do curriculum structures ensure opportunities for developing/enhancing compassion, competence, commitment, conscience, and confidence as expressions of the caring nature of nursing?

- Do course designs and materials foster creativity and responsivity to caring values such as honesty, humility, and multiple ways of knowing?

- Is there evidence that the shared study of nursing articulates nursing as it is understood by nurses practicing in the local and larger community? by persons seeking nursing services?

- Are all relevant constituent groups offered opportunity to explore these questions and have their responses valued?

- Is the curriculum itself valued and prized as enduring and unfolding, all at once?

Following is a range of examples of course assignments and graded activities that illustrate the faculty's commitment to the caring-based transformation of the curriculum. These examples are part of the material studied in the curriculum portion of the overall program evaluation.

Master's Program Comprehensive Exam; Sample Questions.

Example 1. Discuss your concept of advanced nursing practice from the perspective of nursing as promoting the process of being and becoming through caring. Use a nursing situation as the context for your discussion. Choose one general nursing theory to use for comparison, and discuss similarities and differences in advanced nursing practice from the two perspectives.

Example 2. How does your grounding in caring serve as a moral base for advanced nursing practice? Use a nursing situation to illustrate your response. Support your answer with reference to specific nursing literature.

Example 3.   Discuss qualitative and quantitative approaches to nursing inquiry in relation to your understanding of nursing as promoting the process of being and becoming through caring. Include several examples of problems for nursing inquiry to illustrate your discussion.

NUR 4827 Introduction to Professional Nursing Practice.

In the final undergraduate course before graduating, students are asked to write an "initiative letter" to an individual, group, or agency in which they state a personal concern relating to the administration of nursing services in a health care delivery system. One parameter on which the project is evaluated is the extent to which it reflects the course goal related to creating caring environments.

NUR 4296 Issues in Gerontological Nursing.

In this undergraduate elective course, students are free to invite an older adult, with whom they have been meeting, to be with them in the classroom as an expression of the mutuality of the relationship. This is an open invitation, not an assignment.

NUR 3115 Introduction to Nursing as a Discipline and Profession.

Project: Aesthetic Expression of Journey

The purpose of this project is to aesthetically express your journey as a nursing student since enrolling in NUR 3115. Reflect on your journey; select a symbol or metaphor alive with meaning for you, and translate it into an aesthetic expression. Include these elements:

1. Aesthetic expression of journey (a) is unique to nurse person, and (b) reflects special characteristics (background, interests, talents, priorities, and so on) that nurse person brings to situation.

2. Creation or selection (a) points to something greater than itself and (b) has embedded meaning.

3. Creativity is evidenced and might be reflected in imagination; values; assertiveness; playing for keeps; risk taking; glimpses of something one had never thought of, perceived, done, or felt before; attraction to puzzling things; respect for an entire event or recovery of preconscious aspects.

4. Aesthetics is evidenced and might be in keeping with the creation and/or appreciation of a singular, particular, subjective expression of imagined possibilities or equivalent realities that resist projection into the discursive form of language.

One faculty member created a "clinical worksheet" to guide student learning in NUR 4535L, Nursing Situations Lab in Mental Health Settings. This worksheet is completed at the end of each clinical experience. Its purpose, like that of the more traditional "teaching care plan," is to help students recall and integrate their daily experience as part of their growing understanding of nursing. Questions addressed on the worksheet are:

1. Describe the process of being and becoming through caring in the person who is the client. Who is the person and what was the meaning for him or her of the nursing situation?

2. What was the call for nursing? Describe what the client did, said, or was, that prompted you to respond.

3. *Creating the experience of caring.* Identify the

    a. Personal knowing: describe how you felt about yourself—your own feelings, reactions, and behaviors within this nursing situation.

    b. Aesthetic knowing: describe how caring was expressed between the nurse and client. Describe how your care was given and how the client responded to your care.

    c. Empirical knowing: identify new knowledge gained in preparation for and living of this nursing situation.

    d. Ethical knowing: analyze issues and choices that were made in this nursing situation—values, standards, and legal considerations.

4. Identify how the caring between the nurse and client promoted well-being.

Faculty value the insights that students bring to the study of nursing. One student's work, "Pick" (see below), was a response to a journaling assignment following an experience of studying nursing practice in a child care center for disadvantaged children. An aesthetic rendering of a nursing situation from NUR 3116, General Nursing Situations, "Pick" was used by the faculty the next year, for the final examination in the same course. Students were asked to read the nursing situation and respond in an essay to questions about: knowing the person as caring; discussing calls for nursing and nursing responses; material from foundational courses drawn on in studying the situation; and the four patterns of knowing. The nursing situation and selected student responses to the exam questions are reproduced here, to help the reader understand how nursing is being studied in the program.

PICK

"Pick," she said.
"Just pick anyone," she repeated with the casualness of
picking fruit at the fruitstand.
I stared at a deep sea of young faces.
"Pick," I said to myself as the uneasiness of long ago
childhood crept over me.
Oh, the days of being picked last in P.E.
Oh, the fear of being picked first for a spelling bee.
I picked. He was a roly-poly shaggy boy. He talked
fast. He moved fast.
He moved through our time with the speed of lightning;
every moment being seized upon before moving on to the
other.
Though he appeared to me as person, I could not know him.
He would not look me in the eye.
But, who am I to ask this privilege of him? We are
strangers caught in a time and place not of our choosing.
As our time together grew, our outer selves faded away.
He looked within me and knew he could just be . . . and I
could just be. He called to me

for listening
for acceptance
for being
for being free to be himself.

We journeyed through his fast moving maze of Nintendo and
Ninja Turtles, mothers and grandmothers, of God and
spaceships and heaven and Halloween.
And back to earth again.
Our time together was over.
We picked up our outer selves as if they were coats
hanging in a cloakroom. We moved back into our former
spaces and became students once again. A large frown
came over his entire face as he shuffled back to the
classroom.

by Carol Bruce

137

Exam Question 1. Communicate *your* knowing of J. as person uniquely living caring moment-to-moment and expressing his hopes and dreams for growing in caring . . .

Sample Responses:

> This unique remarkable young man exhibits many caring ingredients. He shows honesty and courage—he is willing to know himself and communicate self with others such as the nursing student. J. accepts himself in the moment. He shows patience—not by complacently waiting for life to come to him, but by being open to emerging possibilities, and actively anticipating his own hopes and dreams. I also see alternating rhythms in this lived dialogue. He is at first unwilling to look C. in the eye but later calls to her to join him on his journey. I see J. living caring moment-to-moment in his vibrancy. He appreciates details, whether it be spending time with his family members or playing a game of Nintendo.
>
> ———
>
> J. is a second-grade student who was chosen by a student nurse as her client. At first meeting, this plump, messy, and perhaps typically hyperactive little boy seemed shy, but as the two students began to spend more time with each other, he gave her the privilege of knowing him— eventually their eyes connected. John felt comfortable with her—through his trust—as he felt her acceptance of him. He chattered and chattered with rapid fire as he sensed her desire to listen. He exalted in her presence as she let him be—as she let him be free to be himself.

Exam Question 2. What call for caring does J. communicate most vividly to you? What is one caring response you would like to make . . .

Sample Responses:

I see many calls in this situation, but the most vivid call is that J. is asking for someone to share things with—to pay attention and to accept him. I will be happy to listen to and encourage his ideas about spaceships and Halloween, and let him know how very important and valid these thoughts are. I want to make J. feel good about being himself. I hear a call to encourage J. to celebrate his own being and becoming! This vibrant child is inviting me to explore his hopes and dreams by marveling with him at all the exciting things in his eight-year-old world. I would enjoy participating in J's fast-paced life. I want to encourage his honesty, courage, and trust by supporting and accepting him the way he is, not trying to impose my views onto him. I want to nurture his patience by helping him seek out his future. I want to provide myself to him as a sounding board; one who will encourage him to explore.

———

J's call for nursing, as their eyes connected, was one of trust and patience—to allow him the freedom to be himself. The nursing response is one of listening, assurance, and acceptance through gentle touch and voice—one of gentleness—to nurture J's being.

Exam Question 3.
List at least five points of relevant information from your foundational course work that contributes to your knowing J. in his being and becoming through caring . . .

Sample Responses:

In Psychology class I learned according to Erikson that, as an eight-year-old, J. is struggling between feelings of industry and inferiority. Going to school, away from the family for the first time, he is learning how to be competent at different things as well as learning how to act within a peer group. I can help nurture feelings of competency. In my Growth and Development class I learned about Sameroff's Transactional Model. Development is a result of a continuous interchange between J. and his changing environment. This underscores J's being and all the innumerable, potential "becomings" within J. Also from G&D [Growth and Development], I know that John is in Piaget's Concrete Operations stage. This tells me that J. has the ability to think logically. He understands things like conservation and reversibility. He is able to take another's views into account and is able to converse *with* me, not just *to* me about his dreams. In NUR 3115 we first learned about entering the world of the other for the purpose of knowing the other as caring person. I have never been an eight-year-old boy. In order to see him as caring person, I must put aside my biases and view the world as he views it. As a boy, J. probably participates in more rough-and-tumble play, he is more likely to be aggressive, and he is a bigger risk taker than girls his age. This information from G&D helps me to know him as unique person, and enter his world.

————

The following are relevant statements from course work which contribute to knowing J.:

Caring as a holistic concept (*ANS*, 1990, Concept of Caring).

Authentic presence and angular view (Paterson & Zderad; NUR 3115 Intro to Nursing as a Discipline and Profession)

Being more—to grow from one experience to the next experience (Paterson & Zderad; NUR 3115 Intro to Nursing as Discipline & Profession)

We can understand based only on our own experiences (NUR 3116 General Nursing Situations)

Enable the other to grow in their own time and in their own way (Mayeroff, *On Caring*)

Nursing's goal is to listen and learn what it is to be . . . to promote the process of being and becoming through caring (General Nursing Situations, FAU College of Nursing Philosophy)

Nurses do not "fix" things (General Nursing Situations)

The spirit of nursing to create the availability of freedom of choice (*Holistic Nursing Practice*, 1989, Spirit of Nursing)

Reciprocity, the giving and taking of the nurse and client in a mutually positive way to nurture each other, occurs greatly through the use of intuition (*ANS*, 1990, Therapeutic Reciprocity)

Exam Question 4. . . . detail your knowledge base for the response you proposed in Question 2 . . . address personal, empirical, ethical, and aesthetic patterns of knowing . . . include at least three current sources from nursing journals.

Sample Responses:

Carper's four ways of knowing come alive in this nursing situation with J.

I bring forth empirical knowledge to this situation that helps me know J. First, I have learned a framework by which to identify J. as caring person. This framework assists me in recognizing and answering J's calls for caring. I also have a knowledge base from years (and years and years!) of education. This knowledge, some of which was discussed in Question 3, gives me a *general* background about what to expect from an eight-year-old boy. For instance, I can foresee J. to be struggling with issues of industry versus inferiority. This underscores the call for me to give him my undivided attention, and help him see himself as a worthy, competent individual. The highest-ranked caring behavior Wolfe identifies is "attentive listening." This empirical fact reaffirms what I see as the most vivid call from J.

My ethical knowing of this nursing situation is related to more empirical data. Young children are very impressionable. This knowledge warns me to be extremely careful about not imposing my views on J. about such delicate topics as religion. Bishop and Scudder believe it is imperative that nurses foster the moral autonomy of their clients. I must assist and encourage J. through his exploration of heaven and God, yet I must take care not to lead him in the direction which I have deemed appropriate for myself. This relates to personal knowing, because I must carefully define my own religious opinions to myself in order to be cautious about imposing my personal views onto J. My own value system must be kept separate from his.

Personal knowing is a critical component in this nursing experience. I must continually be re-evaluating myself in order to enter into this situation with authentic presence. This includes recognizing my weaknesses. I have not spent very much time with young children; if I am not careful, there is a good chance that I will communicate my uneasiness at this unfamiliar situation to J. I must consciously look past this unfamiliarity to see J. as caring person, not as just a roly-poly second grader who I don't know what to say to. Here is a person with courage and honesty and trust. I must recognize that J. has calls for caring, and, in turn, J. has much to teach me.

142

This leads me to appreciate the esthetics of this situation. From the little time that I have spent with children, I know that their visions and ideas can be both beautiful and refreshing. Having a chance to experience J's fast-paced world is something I look forward to. This makes me think of Marck's article about therapeutic reciprocity. J. and I both will find empowerment within our unique relationship. J's spirit has so much to teach me! I will draw strength from his vitality and curiosity. He will flourish with the help of my undivided attention. We both will grow in caring.

———

Personal (through centering, intuition and trust). Raising two children of my own would initially aid me in feeling comfortable around J. My previous work in a Day Care Center also gave me insight into what to expect and something to relate this experience to. My personal experience says I would use patience to care for J.

Esthetics (whole picture of knowing—the art).
My mask must crumble—
for me to care for John through knowing—

to use knowledge I know to be true
and knowledge I understand to be true—
the heart will interrelate.
> Our eyes connected
> His touch accepted
> My mind says to care
> My heart tells me how.

Ethical (guide to appropriate action). Before entering into John's situation, I felt I needed to set aside any preconceived ideas I may have on children—once again my mask must crumble. For me to see J. as a unique person, I had to clear my mind.

Empirical (facts, technical aspects). To enhance my physical assessment skills of the child, I would revisit the chapters in Bates (1991) and Bowers et al. (1988). This would give me more confidence in my technical skills. To constantly tune my caring skill, I would also revisit Mayeroff (1971) on trust and patience because I believe these two ingredients of caring were John's main call for nursing. In addition, reviewing Wolfe's (1986, *ANS*) top ten characteristics of caring behavior [would] assist in keeping my caring focused.

In the spirit of nursing and in the ordinariness of nursing, J. needed to be himself and it was my responsibility as nurse to allow him to explore this. However, before our encounter ended, I would need to encourage J. to become independent of me. Newman called this the "moving apart" (Newman, 1989, *Holistic Nursing Practice*). J.'s situation is nursing practice in its ordinariness (Taylor, 1992, *ANS*).

One source of evidence of the valuing and prizing of the curriculum comes in the acceptance of our students' work in journals and other forums. A course assignment in NUR 4746, Nursing Situations in Acute Settings: Adult—to submit for publication papers based on nursing situations experienced in that semester—resulted in three students' papers being published in *Imprint,* the journal of the National Student Nurses Association. A project from NUR 4605, one of the undergraduate nursing practice courses designed specifically for registered nurse students, was presented at a national conference on nursing theory and was subsequently published as a chapter in *Patterns of Nursing Theories in Practice.* Graduate student work has been accepted for presentation at international, national, and regional refereed nursing conferences and published in proceedings.

A stated goal of the master's program refers to preparing students for doctoral study. One master's graduate expressed valuing and prizing the program and her own growth in relation to this goal as follows:

> I graduated from an AAS nursing program in 1964 and have for most of the subsequent time practiced nursing. I have always practiced with a deliberate, thoughtful intention of being the best I could for nursing, described by Styles as personalizing my position within the profession. I have had a full participation in the educational resources of the profession and gave back to the profession my knowing.
>
> I have always had the patient as the focus of my practice and thoughtfully and intentionally searched for (and found) the blessed soul of the other. For me, the patient has always been a reflection of the goodness of the universe and beyond.
>
> I have been blessed with these qualities and the spirit to want to live them to the fullest.
>
> When I came to this master's program I thought I knew nursing and the persons I have nursed. And I did know a lot. However, what was missing from my practice was the ideology of nursing as a discipline of scholars, deliberate attention to knowing nursing more fully by continuously studying, inquiring, sciencing about what it means to nurse the other. And who is this other? Is it really an other or part of the whole? The courage of the scholar to set aside the "here it is, this is all you need to know" and to ask "what if?" and "I think." "Let me share my thoughts with you, let me present my thinking at a conference, let me write this stuff for others to be stimulated to think about" are now emerging and shaky hallmarks of my more fully developing understanding of what it means to be me and nurse.

> I have not only been welcomed into the discipline of scholars at FAU but I have been mentored, nourished, and nurtured in an atmosphere of unending supportive anticipation of my being and becoming.

Employers of the alumni of the program participate in the program evaluation process. On a regular basis, the employers of graduates from one and five years past are asked to provide input on graduates' performance relative to program objectives. In addition, informal opportunities occur for this input. For example, at a regional meeting of nursing leaders from education and service, one director of a hospital nursing service offered her thoughts. She related that FAU graduates do seem different, and when asked to elaborate, she said, "They are so ethically grounded."

An alumna of the undergraduate program offered a story to illustrate her first year of practice and then discussed the impact of the program on her personally and professionally:

> Another patient called me because he was having difficulty breathing. As I entered the room he was sitting up in his bed. I sat down beside him and asked him if sitting up helped him. He said, "Not yet." I asked him to sit up straight and take deep breaths in through his nose and out through his mouth. My patient was watching the weather report on TV where a hurricane was being discussed. I asked my patient if he was tracking the hurricane. He said that he was and told me about being in the hurricane in Miami. I said it must have been a scary time. And we sat and talked about his experience. His breath seemed to improve and I asked him if it had. He said he was breathing better and laid back down in his bed. He thanked me for sitting with him. I told him he was welcome and if he had any more problems to call me right away. I could see the relief in his face.

I had the opportunity to go to two different nursing schools. The first was an excellent school and basically focused on technical skills. We had a philosophy; however, we really didn't incorporate it into the program.

FAU was a very different program. In the beginning, it was very difficult to understand and I didn't know how to incorporate the philosophy into practice. As much as I hated journaling, I believe it helped me a great deal in learning myself and my patients. Because of journaling I was able to know my feelings and values. I realized that if I didn't know myself, it would be impossible to know and understand my patients.

I can see a very big difference in how I practice nursing and how other nurses practice. As a graduate of a caring-based program I feel caring is not taken for granted. It's always in the forefront. Caring is an art and I believe FAU's philosophy brought the art of nursing into my practice.

Following completion of a graduate elective course, NGR 6930, Nursing Education Centered in Caring, a graduate student and long-time faculty member in an associate degree nursing program wrote of her growing in caring:

Once upon a time there was a nurse who thought that she taught nursing to beginning students. She spent much of her career in nursing as an instructor, and although she knew that she sincerely cared about the nursing students and did her very best to help them learn about nursing and what it means to be a nurse, she one day discovered how very much more she could help them. She had always believed that caring, compassion, and patience were essential components of nursing, and did her best to live out these qualities with patients and with the nursing students. She very much believed that nursing students learned many of what she considered to be the real fundamentals of nursing through a process of role modeling, and so tried to live these qualities in all areas of her life as an instructor of nursing.

The instructor decided to go back to school and further her study of nursing. She was exposed to a caring-based nursing program that validated so many of her beliefs and helped to describe so much of what she felt in nursing. She came to realize how very committed she was to the discipline of nursing and how very valuable the profession of nursing was to her. New doors were opened for her as she listened to others who articulated what she felt. A basic assumption of the caring-based program is that all persons are caring, in that caring is the human mode of being. This framework supported the basic personal and professional beliefs of the instructor, and she found herself very much at peace within this program.

Once the instructor attended a week-long class on nursing education centered in caring. Through the readings, and dialogue of the group, she came to understand new ways of teaching and understanding the discipline and profession of nursing. She realized that so much of what she taught was from the discipline of medicine rather than nursing, and learned to understand and value the importance of distinguishing the two disciplines. She came to see how nursing stories of nursing situations could express the essence of nursing. She realized that some of her favorite "lectures" of the past were ones in which she shared personal nursing stories with the students. Looking back, she had known that students learn best when they can relate something to a person. Looking forward, she knew that nursing is being with persons, nurturing their being and becoming through caring, and that this is not something of nursing or in nursing, but it *is* nursing. She knew that the value of these stories is that they speak, and describe the artful

148

science of nursing, a discipline inclusive of personal, empirical, ethical, and aesthetic knowledge. She knew that taking this class had especially opened her eyes to the value of aesthetic expression in nursing education. From then on, she knew that she could teach nursing, and she knew what nursing is.

STUDENTS

The evaluation of student learning in a caring-based program must begin with the student and the faculty knowing self and other as caring person. This is the orienting position, which ensures that evaluation will be a process of valuing, prizing, and growing. The faculty role in evaluating student learning is twofold, in concert with the student's simultaneous objectives of learning and having that learning warranted as academic credit. The terms *formative* (growth-promoting) and *summative* (grade award) are sometimes used to convey this dualistic emphasis. The faculty values both the distinction and the interrelation between formative and summative evaluation. The purpose for which the decision is being made guides the choice of summative versus formative perspective; however, the view of persons being and becoming through caring requires that there be a formative element in any summative evaluation. This translates into the understanding that, in all situations, a deliberate emphasis is on knowing and affirming self and other as caring persons unfolding possibilities for expressing caring in new ways.

Does the commitment to a caring-based program mean that the faculty project no expectations, that standards are nonexistent or soft, that "anything goes?" By no means. The faculty as avowed members of the discipline value and prize the idea of nursing and the studied practice of nursing, and work diligently to communicate caring as they live out their teaching role in ways that demonstrate these ideals. Further, the service nature of nursing calls for unambiguous and lofty standards. It is precisely the commitment to the value of persons being and becoming through caring that enables faculty to assist students to embrace high standards in the study of nursing. The faculty expect students to explore and to create personal ways of effectively expressing nursing. There is an effort in each course—and even in each clinical or classroom period—to keep in mind that summative determinations come at the end of the course, not the beginning or the middle.

Course objectives are expressions of the faculty's understanding of the course in relation to other courses and to the program. Course objectives for all courses are specific applications of overall program objectives and are derived from the major themes of the conceptual framework (itself an expression of the philosophy of the program). This close correspondence between program objectives and course objectives is a deliberate effort to ensure coherence, rather than adherence. Course objectives are broadly drawn—again, deliberately—to permit uniqueness and creativity within a stable but evolving understanding of the nature and content of the discipline. These objectives serve as guides to teaching/learning in a particular course and also as standards for evaluation. Objectives at all levels of the graduate and undergraduate programs reflect the themes of the organizing framework: images of nurse and nursing; nursing as a discipline; nursing as a profession; person being and becoming through caring; and nursing as promoting the process of being and becoming through caring.

Rather than going back to tortuous and, we believe, ultimately trivializing efforts at quantification (e.g., behavioral objectives), the faculty's sense of entry and exit expectations for each course is communicated more qualitatively—in the particular emphasis evident in objectives from one course to another, in the details of assignments, and in the discussion of expectations regarding assignments. Journaling assignments are a good example of how students are encouraged to reflect understanding with increasing depth, scope, and integration. For instance, in the first undergraduate course, students may be asked to keep a journal for reflecting on their being and becoming through caring as beginning students of professional nursing. These students are encouraged to employ the four patterns of knowing in their reflections, to incorporate their experience (past and present), and to draw on at least two scholarly journal articles from a list provided. By contrast, in NGR 5018, Caring: Foundations for Advanced Nursing, the introductory graduate-level nursing course, students are given an appropriately more sophisticated journal assignment. They are asked to keep a journal in which they reflect their growing understanding of caring as the essence of nursing as they dialogue with the authors of six selected readings. Each of these assignments provides a meaningful challenge to growth in nursing, regardless of the level of the program. In keeping with caring values, objectives are viewed by the faculty person as points of orientation rather than as templates for action. This approach requires that faculty, as well as students, are known as caring persons unfolding hopes and dreams. It also requires considerable ongoing dialogue between students and faculty as well as among faculty colleagues.

What happens when, after engaging with students in the study of a particular range of nursing situations over the course of a semester, a faculty member determines that an individual student has not accomplished the objectives of the course? The faculty member as person finds guidance in his or her developed understanding of living caring in the academic setting. The explicit grounding of all persons and activities in a commitment to and knowledge of caring helps to ensure on a consistent basis that individuals are respected and shared social values are honored. Students in a caring-based program can and do fail courses. What is different is how persons are with each other and how they proceed in relationship. Because of the grounding in caring, educational ideals are more consistently approximated—ideals such as the student's having been: carefully advised along the way that a time frame exists, given multiple legitimate opportunities to engage productively with the teacher and other students in the particular learning experiences offered, and advised in a timely fashion that course objectives were not being accomplished at satisfactory levels. When a student fails a course, this needs to be communicated in an environment of continuing to learn, continuing to be known as caring person and person of value. The teacher must strive to enter into the discussion in a spirit of courage, honesty, and humility. Further, the committed faculty person remembers that any engagement with nursing, even such a stressful one, should be an expression of caring. Does this mean that students don't experience the painful shame of failure? No; but the faculty person committed to affirming the other as caring person of value accepts the responsibility to communicate a larger context and to remain available for further growth-promoting opportunities. Legitimate appeal procedures are in place, and there is concerted effort to make students aware of these procedures, both in general orientations and in immediate situations.

In the general format for clinical evaluation of student learning, the set of course objectives is arrayed on one side of the page, with space across from each for writing examples of the student's having achieved/not achieved the objective. At the end, there is a designated space for a summary statement. Both faculty and student fill out this form, at midterm and at the end of the course. In addition, for those courses in which the student studies with a practicing nurse preceptor, the preceptor participates in ongoing and final evaluation of the student's progress in achieving course objectives.

The following final summary evaluation from the beginning undergraduate nursing practice course demonstrates the early emphasis on the student of nursing:

> [Student's name] has demonstrated much growth over the course of the semester. She is able to articulate nursing situations, identify calls for nursing, and respond appropriately. She is able to critically read and select information relevant to the study of particular nursing situations—readings are excellent. Of the patterns of knowing, it appears she struggles most with the ethical knowing but has again grown with this. She is very caring and compassionate. Her "person" reflects sincerity and warmth.

One beginning nursing student evaluated her progress in identifying calls and responses in nursing situations in this way:

> This is probably where I grew the most in this course. I started from scratch as I wasn't sure about the existence of calls from healthy individuals. I learned to recognize subtle calls for listening and encouraging my elderly client, and calls to celebrate the many possibilities of a new child with my pregnant couple. My nurturing responses were varied; for instance, I encouraged my elderly client to continue to knit after her stroke because she was good at it, but she doubted herself. I realized the importance of these quiet calls and recognized that they are a critical part of nursing.

Figure 8–1 illustrates a clinical evaluation form, with stated objectives and midterm and final evaluation comments, for NUR 4255L, Nursing Situations in Acute Settings: Adult.

Figure 8–1
Completed Clinical Evaluation Form

Course Objectives and Behavioral Outcomes	Comments (Midterm)	Comments (Final)
1. Discuss images of nurse and nursing held by participants: a. client of nursing; b. student and practitioner of nursing; c. all others providing direct and indirect service; d. larger community.	[Student's name] has been challenged this semester by a variety of images of nursing and nursing (ICU, telemetry, patients' images).	[Student's name]'s journal reflects a questioning and growth in her personal image of nurse and nursing and in her perception of self as nurse.
2. Demonstrate an integrated understanding of knowledge needed to identify calls for nursing and nursing responses in acute situations.	[Student's name] is consistently unable to identify calls and responses. Her knowledge of pathophysiology needs to increase.	[Student's name]'s abilities to identify calls developed over the course of the semester. She became less focused on tech-technical skills and more open and available to her patients.
3. Demonstrate an integrated understanding of knowledge of professional nursing in acute nursing situations: a. social responsibility and accountability; b. personal and professional leadership; c. values, standards, ethics, and legal systems.	[Student's name] is well prepared for clinicals. Needs to continue to work on pulling the whole nursing situation together.	[Student's name] is consistently well-prepared for clinicals and has demonstrated increased ability to view the nursing situation as a whole instead of discrete separate parts through her journals, group discussions, and dialogue with clinical instructor.

Figure 8–1 *(Continued)*

Course Objectives and Behavioral Outcomes	Comments (Midterm)	Comments (Final)
4. Develop an understanding of the meaning of being and becoming through caring expressed by clients and nurses in calls and responses in nursing situations with adults in acute settings.	[Student's name] demonstrates an understanding of the process of being and becoming through caring that is reflected in the care she provides for her clients and her journal entries. She needs to strive to be more articulate about the process.	[Student's name]'s ability to articulate her understanding of the process of being and becoming through caring has greatly improved. Her journals reflect depth of understanding that she has been able to demonstrate with her interactions with patients and families.
5. Demonstrate an understanding of nursing as the promotion of being and becoming through caring in nursing situations with adults in acute settings.	[Student's name] seeks out challenging nursing situations that will foster her development.	[Student's name] has worked hard this semester to incorporate her clinical skills with psychosocial support in the nursing situations she encountered. She is able to raise significant clinical questions that support and challenge her understanding of promoting the process of being and becoming through caring.

Students receive a letter grade in clinical courses as well as classroom courses—a change that was long studied and discussed within the College of Nursing. The primary rationale for change related to caring: caring for the student and caring for the discipline. Many, although not all, students felt that a grade of "satisfactory" did not reflect their commitment, effort, and accomplishment in clinical learning. In addition, the high number of ungraded credits made nursing students ineligible for honors designations by the University Registrar at graduation. Initially, several members of the faculty advocated this change to reflect the value of excellence in nursing practice. After a four-year period of discussion and experimentation, the faculty adopted the practice of awarding letter grades in clinical courses.

Often, the faculty person invites student input into evaluation parameters for particular assignments, especially in senior and graduate-level courses. For example, in NGR 5018, Caring: Foundation for Advanced Nursing, students were invited to participate in the development of evaluation criteria for a project calling for the aesthetic representation of caring in a nursing situation. This process involved dialogue, over time, so that the process emerging was satisfying to all concerned. Figure 8–2 reproduces the guidelines for an assigned aesthetic project in NUR 3116, General Nursing Situations, along with the format used for evaluating the project. Figure 8–3 shows an example from NGR 5110, Nursing Theories, in which students present theories of nursing and their peers provide an evaluation. The evaluation is given to the presenting student, who uses peer evaluations in preparing a self-evaluation. The self-evaluation is provided to the faculty as input into the 30 percent grade allocation for this assignment.

Figure 8–2
Assignment Guidelines and Evaluation Framework for an
Aesthetic Project in NUR 3116   General Nursing Situations

FLORIDA ATLANTIC UNIVERSITY
COLLEGE OF NURSING

NUR 3116   GENERAL NURSING SITUATIONS
Fall 1991

GUIDELINES FOR AESTHETIC PROJECT

PURPOSE: The purpose of the aesthetic project is to provide the opportunity to express a fully integrated understanding of the concept of a nursing situation: a lived experience in which the caring between nurse and the one nursed promotes well-being.

GUIDELINES: Using any medium of aesthetic expression that you choose, "re-present" a nursing situation of your experience, communicating in that "re-presentation" the sense of a lived experience in which the caring between nurse and the one nursed promotes well-being.

Aesthetic media can take many forms, for example: dance, painting, sketching, photography, theater, song, poetry, three-dimensional art, quilting, embroidery, puppetry, film, sculpture, pottery, and so on.

RECOMMENDATION: Choose a nursing situation that you experienced as a nursing situation this semester. Dwell with that situation and try to get a full sense of that as a lived experience shared by you and your client in which caring developed between you, and the growth that you both experienced in that situation. When you have this sense, then choose an art form to make that situation live anew.

EVALUATION: This is the evaluation form I will use in assigning a grade to the project:

Objective: To represent a nursing situation through an artistic medium.

A   (comprehensive, clear, integrated understanding of outstanding depth demonstrated)

157

Figure 8–2 *(Continued)*

B (depth of comprehension, clarity, and integration of understanding demonstrated)

C (comprehensive, clear, integrated understanding demonstrated)

D Integrated understanding not demonstrated)

Nursing Situation:

Lived Experience:

Caring between nurse and one nursed *promotes well-being:*

Final Project Grade (representation of a lived experience between nurse and the one nursed promotes well-being):

Figure 8–3
Format for Peer Evaluation of Presentation in
NGR 5110   Nursing Theories

FLORIDA ATLANTIC UNIVERSITY
COLLEGE OF NURSING

NGR 5110   NURSING THEORIES
Fall 1993

Student Evaluation of Projects/Presentations

Name of Presenter: _____

Name of Evaluator: _____

Topic: _____

Date: _____

The Project/Presentation was:

    Outstanding   _____
    Very Good   _____
    Satisfactory   _____
    Unsatisfactory _____

Rationale for rating based on purpose and guidelines of the projects: (use additional space as needed)

FACULTY

Formal structures for evaluating faculty include annual evaluation, merit evaluation, and evaluation for tenure and for promotion. College of Nursing faculty have developed the guidelines for these evaluation opportunities, and these guidelines have gained approval of the University Provost. These guidelines are continuously unfolding as the faculty struggles with issues of continuity and creativity in the evolving understanding of the discipline. The development and revision of guidelines is an exercise in caring—caring for the discipline and striving to articulate standards that demonstrate its value in society; caring for persons and striving to demonstrate commitment to the discipline, through teaching, research, and service, in ways that are satisfying to the person and contribute to the advancement of nursing.

Processes and products of constructing guidelines and formats are opportunities to live out caring values, but how persons are with each other in the faculty evaluation process is most important. During evaluation processes, all relevant persons are invited to contribute input, including students, peers, and administrator(s), as well as the person whose work is being reviewed. In meetings where faculty is called on for summative evaluation of peers, the stage needs to be set so that a caring environment—evocative of diverse caring values such as courage, humility, honesty, and multiple ways of knowing—prevails. Again, as with evaluation of students, being part of a caring-based program does not mean that salary increases and tenure awards are guaranteed. Those determinations are made in dialogue, endeavoring to relate previously worked-out and evolving understandings of quality and suitability in unique, particular, personal situations.

In a caring-based program that emphasizes valuing the person and prizing both being and becoming through caring, informal dialogues of "How am I doing? What are you doing?" occur daily. Faculty persons value themselves, their work in nursing education, their colleagues, and their mutual enterprise. Because of the "course-responsible teacher" approach, faculty are not inundated with team or section meetings. It is at the initiative of individual faculty persons that informal dialogues, usually highly spirited and equally profitable, occur—in faculty offices, in the college kitchen, and even in hallways. The values emphasized in a caring-based program minimize competition, give permission for valuing self and one's experimentations, and promote a spirit of curiosity about the discoveries being made by colleagues. At formal and informal gatherings where valuing, prizing, and growing are of concern, there is an effort to remember that faculty are continuously growing in knowing themselves as caring persons, that each of us is at our own point of unfolding in any given moment, and that growing is nurtured in our dialogue.

ADMINISTRATION

The administration of the program, or of various parts of it, is seen as "ministering to" the persons involved in the enterprise, including respecting policies as guidelines operationalizing caring values expressed by the faculty. Administration in a caring-based program is a form of contribution to the circle of caring persons participating in the program.

As with other components of the program, persons are valued, prized, and helped to grow as they minister in the context of particular administrative roles. And, like titles in other program components (such as student, faculty, staff), administrator is the name of a role that highlights certain central functions carried out by the person in the role. At all times, administrator must be known, by self and others, as *person* being and becoming through caring.

Like other components of the program, evaluation of administration occurs both informally and formally. The ideals of persons being known as caring and of openness to dialogue are sources of courage in communicating honestly with persons in administrative roles. All of Mayeroff's caring ingredients are called on when faculty, students, staff, and other administrators approach persons in administrative roles with potentially painful observations, even when the observations are offered in the spirit of facilitating growth. The College of Nursing's tradition of an "open door" policy among administrators invites engagement. Because this policy carries risk, it is a courageous, humble, hopeful expression of caring.

This attitude toward administration and administrators provides direction for relationships with central administrators beyond the College. The President, Provost, and other university executives are seen as dancers in the circle of caring persons committed to the welfare and effectiveness of the College of Nursing.

The formal evaluation plan for the College includes administrator review on a periodic basis. The Dean and Program Directors are evaluated in their roles every 5 years, concurrent with the timetable at the University. The internal review is conducted by the Executive Council of the College. (The Dean does not sit with the Executive Council in these reviews, nor does a Program Director who is being evaluated.) Written input is sought from faculty, students, and staff, as well as from the person being evaluated. Figure 8–4 illustrates the current administrator evaluation form. (The Executive Council from time to time creates additional processes.)

Figure 8–4
Administrator Evaluation Form

FLORIDA ATLANTIC UNIVERSITY
COLLEGE OF NURSING

ADMINISTRATIVE EFFECTIVENESS APPRAISAL

Ratings range from 5 (highest) to 1 (lowest).

1. Has ability and willingness to "open doors" for faculty members.
2. Attends to details effectively.
3. Instills enthusiasm for professional goals.
4. Judges people perceptively and fairly.
5. Keeps abreast of new developments and innovations in higher education.
6. Makes sound decisions.
7. Plans effectively and imaginatively.
8. Resolves or ameliorates human conflicts.
9. Says "no" effectively.
10. Understands and uses modern management procedures.
11. Is willing to appraise situations and problems impartially.
12. Is willing to put others first.
13. Works effectively with faculty members.
14. Works effectively with other administrators.
15. Overall rating:

Input is compiled by the Executive Council and reported at a meeting of the faculty of the College. After dialogue, a report is given by the Executive Council to the Dean. When an administrator other than the Dean is being evaluated, the Dean meets with the person being evaluated, for dialogue.

RESOURCES

The component of resources covers a variety of specific entities. The evaluation plan lists clinical agencies, office space, classrooms, conference rooms, equipment, support services (including clerical staff, student assistants, library, computer services, and student affairs), and instructional materials. Each of these resource areas is recognized as participating in the circle of caring as persons make contributions that forward the goals of the College of Nursing. A spirit of caring needs to prevail as each resource is valued and helped to grow. Evaluation of several of these areas will be addressed for purposes of illustration.

Persons who make up the clerical staff are valued and prized in many ways: by being known as person, by being welcomed into dance of nursing, and by having opportunities to explore personal ways of growing within the context of the organizational framework, and to collaborate in planning work and allocating responsibilities. Periodic meetings are held in which administrators and staff share ideas about the effective functioning of the College and develop plans for ensuring the caring environment.

Practice settings where nursing is studied are selected with care and brought into the dance of nursing. The format used by faculty to record evaluation of clinical agencies at the end of each course is based on the following points:

1. Nature and range of nursing situations within agency.
2. Accomplishment of the objectives at the site.
3. Extent of caring and receptiveness by nurses and personnel.
4. Physical setting (i.e., private, comfortable space for conferences).
5. Consideration for change in setting based on personal input, student input, or agency personnel.
6. Recommendations for change, especially improving relations between agency setting and College of Nursing/FAU.

These formal evaluations generally take place at the end of each course, sometimes at meetings with nurse managers from all relevant areas and all nursing faculty who used the setting.

In summary, evaluation is understood to be a process of caring, a process that focuses on valuing, prizing, and growing. In living this process, faculty, students, and members of the university and larger community come together to acknowledge and affirm nursing. Evaluation is part of the dance of caring persons in the circle of nursing.

Past and Present Faculty Contributors

Cathy Appleton
Linda Beaulieu
Cheryl Beck
Anita Beckerman
Judy Best-Haley
Evelyn Bohm
Anne Boykin
Nancie Bruce
Carolyn Burr
Grace Cattell
Susan Chase
Sherrilyn Coffman
Jessie Colin
Tawna Cooksey
Diane Cope
Sue Doody
Patricia Evans

Susan Folden
Shirley Gordon
Elise Gropper-Katz
Lorranie Haertel
Kathleen Kelley
Lois Kelley
Deirdre Krause
Rozzano Locsin
Donna Maheady
Kathleen Mele
Patricia Munhall
Cheryl Naples
Barbara Nash
Lois Nelson
Danette Ouellette
Lynn Palma
Marilyn Parker

Living a Caring-Based Program

Linda Pumpian
Marilyn Ray
Jdee Richardson
Mary Ellen Robertson
Savina Schoenhofer
Eleanor Schuster
Carol Shimer
Patricia Siccardi

Evelyn Singer
Theresa Simpson
Mary Tarson
Sara Torres
Terri Touhy
Cathie Wallace
Marguerita Warner
Jill Winland-Brown

Courses in Curriculum

Undergraduate

NSP 3185   **Personal Decision-Making for Wellness**
The philosophical and historical aspects of wellness are explored, and the wellness concepts foundational to caring for self are studied.

NSP 3186   **Strategies for Personal Wellness**
Selected wellness appraisal and enhancement strategies are studied, with an emphasis on application.

NUR 3065   **Modes of Helping I**
Focuses on skills necessary for holistic assessment, including history taking, physical assessment, and basic communication skills.

NUR 3065L   **Modes of Helping Lab I**
Acquisition of holistic assessment skills in laboratory setting.

NUR 3106   **Modes of Helping II**
Guided learning of selected technological skills in campus and clinical laboratory settings, based on knowledge of scientific principles.

NUR 3115   **Introduction to Nursing as a Discipline and Profession**
An introduction to nursing as a distinct discipline of knowledge and a unique professional service. Concepts introduced in this course are foundational to the program and include: Images of the nurse and nursing; nursing as a discipline of knowledge; nursing as a profession; being and becoming through caring; and nursing as the promotion of the process of being and becoming through caring.

NUR 3116   **General Nursing Situations**
Study of general nursing situations with individuals of all ages.

NUR 3116L   **General Nursing Situations Lab**
Clinical study of general nursing situations with individuals of all ages.

NUR 3126   **Pathophysiology I**

NUR 3127   **Pathophysiology II**
Study of pathologic alterations in psychologic and biologic subsystems that influence health state in individual human systems.

170

Nonpathologic alterations that have implications for human system patterning, such as pregnancy, are also examined. Diagnostic and medical treatment modalities are studied in conjunction with alterations. A two-course series.

NUR 3745   **Nursing Situations in Acute Settings: Parents and Children**
Study of nursing situations in acute hospital settings that focus on persons of parents and children.

NUR 3455L   **Nursing Situations Lab in Childbearing Settings**
Clinical study of nursing situations that focus on persons involved in childbearing.

NUR 3356L   **Nursing Situations Lab in Acute Settings: Children**
Clinical study of nursing situations that focus on children in acute hospital settings.

NUR 4746   **Nursing Situations in Acute Settings: Adult**
Study of nursing situations in acute hospital settings that focus on adult persons.

NUR 4255L   **Nursing Situations Lab in Acute Settings: Adult**
Clinical study of nursing situations in acute hospital settings that focus on adult persons.

NUR 4535L   **Nursing Situations Lab**
Clinical study of nursing situations that focus on persons in mental health settings.

NUR 4165   **Nursing Research**
Focuses on research as an essential component of nursing as a professional system.
Relationships among theory development, research, and the practice of nursing are examined. Knowledge and skills necessary for
critical analysis of conceptual and technical
aspects of research reports are emphasized.

NUR 4635   **Nursing Situations in the Community:
Families/Groups**
Study of nursing situations in the community, with a focus on persons in families and
groups.

NUR 4635L   **Nursing Situations in the Community:
Families/Groups Lab**
Clinical study of nursing situations in the
community, with a focus on persons in
families and groups.

NUR 4747   **Nursing Situations in Home and Rehabilitation Settings**
Study of nursing situations in the community, in the home, and in rehabilitation
settings.

NUR 4748L   **Nursing Situations Lab: Rehabilitation Settings**
Clinical study of nursing situations of persons in rehabilitation settings.

NUR 4749L   **Nursing Situations Lab: Long-Term
and Home Settings**
Clinical study of nursing situations of persons in long-term and home settings.

NUR 4827 **Introduction to Professional Nursing Practice**
The focus of this course is on the study of the full scope of beginning professional nursing practice.

NUR 4827L **Introduction to Professional Nursing Practice Lab**
The focus of this course is on the clinical study of the full scope of beginning professional nursing practice.

NUR 4605 **Nursing Situations: Healthy Individuals, Families, and Groups**
Study of nursing situations involving healthy individuals, families, and groups in the community. Enrollment limited to professional nurses.

NUR 4605L **Nursing Situations: Healthy Individuals, Families, and Groups Lab**
Clinical study of nursing situations involving healthy individuals, families, and groups in the community. Enrollment limited to professional nurses.

NUR 4606 **Nursing Situations: Individuals, Families, and Groups with a Health Alteration**
Study of nursing situations involving individuals, families, or groups experiencing a crisis, loss, or long-term health alterations. Enrollment limited to professional nurses.

NUR 4606L   **Nursing Situations: Individuals, Families, and Groups with a Health Alteration Lab**

Clinical study of nursing situations involving individuals, families, or groups experiencing crisis, loss, or long-term health alterations. Enrollment limited to professional nurses.

NUR 4296   **Gerontological Nursing Issues**

Approaching aging from a humanistic and holistic perspective, the course focus is on increasing awareness of personal and professional feelings about aging, exploring significant issues in care of the older adult, and developing a professional stance that reflects commitment to promotion of wellness in an aging society.

NUR 4137   **High-Risk Parenting: Nursing Assessment and Strategies**

The focus is on the concept of high-risk parenting through a presentation of the most common high-risk conditions confronting nursing. An understanding of the holistic approach to patient care is developed by examination of nursing assessment and strategies.

NUR 4495   **Issues in Women's Health Care**

Traditional and nontraditional strategies in the prevention and management of common health alterations of women will be explored. Physiological and psychosocial responses to such alterations will be examined. Students will examine varying viewpoints related to contemporary issues and concerns in gyneco-logical and reproductive health care.

NUR 4823   **Ethics in Nursing**
Basic theories of moral development will be presented. Stages of moral judgment in Kohl-berg's Theory of Moral Development will be examined in relation to the range of re-sponses nurses make to ethical dilemmas. Nursing responsibilities in ethical dilemmas will be analyzed.

NUR 4595   **Women, Witches, and Healing**
A consideration of the nature of wholeness, health, and healing from philosophical, his-torical, cultural, ecological, and feminist per-spectives. The role of healer is visited, especially in relation to contemporary and future professional nursing. Past and current misconceptions and issues are identified and explored.

NUR 3075   **Nursing with Cross-Cultural Child-bearing Families**
Nursing care of the childbearing families from different cultures.

Graduate

NGR 5018   **Caring: Foundation for Advanced Nursing**
A detailed examination of caring as the es-sential concept for nursing knowledge and practice.

NGR 5110   **Nursing Theories**
Nursing models and theories are analyzed as the basis for nursing practice.

NGR 5700   **Creative Leadership in Nursing**
An examination of strategies essential to leadership in nursing and an exploration of creative approaches used to influence health care at all levels.

NGR 5810   **Advanced Nursing Research Methods**
Discusses the relationship on inquiry, including quantitative and qualitative processes, to the advancement and structuring of nursing knowledge.

NGR 6200   **Advanced Nursing: Healthy Adult**
Examines current nursing and nursing-related knowledge as bases for advanced nursing practice with healthy adults. Combines nursing theories, research strategies, ways of knowing and caring, and wellness issues in advanced nursing practice.

NGR 6210   **Advanced Nursing: Adult with Acute and Complex Needs**
Examines current nursing and nursing-related knowledge as bases for advanced nursing practice with adults who have acute and complex needs. Combines nursing theories, research strategies, and ways of knowing and caring with current health issues and advanced nursing practice.

NGR 6630 **Advanced Nursing: Healthy Family**
Examines current nursing and nursing-related knowledge as bases for advanced nursing practice with healthy families.

NGR 6632 **Advanced Nursing: Troubled Families**
Examines current nursing and nursing-related knowledge as bases for advanced nursing practice with families experiencing challenging health situations.

NGR 6720 **Advanced Nursing: Nursing Administration**
Concepts pertinent to the administration of nursing services are examined.

NGR 6725 **Advanced Nursing: Strategies of Nursing Administration**
Detailed processes of nursing management are examined.

NGR 6932 **Advanced Nursing: Adult Seminar**
A forum to discuss nursing issues relevant to advanced nursing practice with adults.

NGR 6936 **Advanced Nursing: Family Seminar**
A forum to discuss nursing issues relevant to advanced nursing practice with families.

NGR 6937 **Introduction to Advanced Nursing Practice: Seminar**
Provides students with the opportunity to discuss the application of advanced knowledge of caring, research, nursing theory, leadership, and knowledge from supporting courses to general nursing situations.

NGR 6938   **Advanced Nursing Research Methods Seminar**
A forum for discussion of the development, application, and evaluation of various types of nursing research.

NGR 6939   **Advanced Nursing: Nursing Administration Seminar**
A forum for students to discuss issues relevant to the practice of nursing administration and to explore creative ways to integrate advanced nursing and supporting knowledge in administration of nursing services.

NGR 6940   **Advanced Nursing: Adult Practicum**
An application of advanced nursing and supporting knowledge in nursing practice with adults.

NGR 6941   **Introduction to Advanced Nursing Practice: Practicum**
A clinical practicum that provides students the opportunity to apply advanced nursing knowledge of caring, research, nursing theory, and leadership in general nursing situations.

NGR 6942   **Advanced Nursing: Family Practicum**
An application of advanced nursing and supporting knowledge in nursing practice with families.

NGR 6943   **Advanced Nursing: Nursing Administration Practicum**
Application of advanced nursing and supporting knowledge in the practice of nursing administration.

NGR 6970   **Project**

An opportunity to develop and pursue a scholarly project other than a thesis. A project is a form of systemic investigation that results in a creative product reflecting in-depth understanding and representation of an aspect of nursing knowledge. A total of 5 credits is required for project completion.

NGR 6971   **Research Thesis**

The design and implementation of a formal research project. A total of 5 credits is required for thesis completion.

Undergraduate Program: Purpose and Objectives

The purpose of the College of Nursing is congruent with the mission of Florida Atlantic University, which is to provide a well-rounded education to its culturally and ethnically diverse student population, with emphasis on the ability to think critically, to operate from an ethical base, and to contribute creatively to a rapidly changing world.

The purpose of the undergraduate nursing program is to prepare the baccalaureate professional nurse generalist to assume beginning roles in the provision of professional nursing to individuals and groups in a variety of settings. Inherent in this central purpose is the intent to provide the foundation for continued study of nursing at the master's level and for advancement to nursing positions of increasing responsibility and leadership. To these ends, the program intends to ensure that the university-educated nurse who graduates from this program has acquired the essential elements of general education as defined by the faculty of Florida Atlantic University and the initial professional education necessary for the practice of nursing. The undergraduate nursing major is concentrated at the upper division level. The nursing program builds on general education courses in the lower division and includes upper-division courses selected from the sciences, arts, and humanities. The education program for professional nursing intends to prepare individuals to make and act on sound judgments using knowledge of the social and natural sciences and the humanities and of professional nursing. The educational program further intends to assist individuals to develop and express caring as a fundamental human characteristic and as essential for professional nursing.

The upper-division nursing program is designed to assist students to gain knowledge of the theory and practice of nursing. The program aims to prepare a practitioner who promotes the process of being and becoming through caring with individuals, families, and groups within communities and societies. The program is designed to emphasize nursing as a discipline of knowledge and a field of professional practice. Emphasis is also placed on collaboration with colleagues in nursing and other health care disciplines in the advancement of understanding and betterment of personal and communal living within a global environment.

The graduate of the program will:

1. Create patterns of nursing that promote the process of being and becoming through caring and express this focus as a generalist in nursing practice.

2. Use personal, empirical, ethical, and aesthetic patterns of knowing in the practice of nursing.

3. Demonstrate social responsibility and accountability as a member of the nursing profession.

4. Exercise personal and professional leadership in the promotion of caring environments.

5. Use systematic inquiry to make beginning contributions to the body of nursing knowledge.

6. Collaborate with colleagues in nursing and other health care disciplines and consumers to promote the well-being and becoming of society.

7. Have a foundation for advanced study in nursing.

Graduate Program: Purpose and Objectives

The purpose of the graduate program is to prepare university-educated registered nurses to assume advanced roles in nursing practice with adults and families and in the beginning practice of nursing administration. This purpose includes the intent of providing the foundation for doctoral-level study in nursing. The program of graduate study is built on the foundation of the undergraduate program and emphasizes the advanced study of nursing as promotion of the process of being and becoming through caring. Graduate study is organized into two levels: (1) core and (2) area of concentration. The purpose of the core is to develop advanced knowledge and understanding of general concepts foundational to the discipline and practice of nursing. These concepts include caring, theory and research, creative leadership, and the practice of nursing. The purpose of the area of concentration is to develop detailed knowledge of a specific field of nursing, integrated into the framework of understanding gained in the core, providing the basis for advanced practice in specific ranges of nursing situations and roles. These areas of concentration include nursing of adults, nursing of families, and nursing administration. A further purpose of the graduate program is to prepare persons who are committed to the advancement of the discipline of nursing and to excellence in nursing practice and who have the knowledge and skills necessary to actualize that commitment.

The graduate of the program will:

1. Create advanced patterns of nursing that promote being and becoming through caring and express this focus in advanced nursing roles.

2. Use nursing theory as a basis for advanced nursing practice.

3. Conduct systematic investigations for the advancement of nursing as a discipline and profession.

4. Influence the well-being and becoming of persons, families, groups, communities, and societies through caring relationships and interrelationships with the environment.

5. Demonstrate expertise in a specialized area of nursing.

6. Have a foundation for doctoral study and continued professional development.

Other Books of Interest from NLN Press

You may order NLN books by ● TELEPHONE 800-NOW-9NLN, ext. 138
● FAX 212-989-3710 ● MAIL Simply use the order form below

Book Title	Pub. No.	Price	NLN Member Price
☐ Nursing As Caring: A Model for Transforming Practice *By Anne Boykin & Savina Schoenhofer*	15-2549	$35.95	$30.95
☐ Nursing Research: A Qualitative Perspective *By Patricia L. Munhall & Carolyn Oiler Boyd*	19-2535	35.95	31.95
☐ Patterns of Nursing Theories in Practice *Edited by Marilyn E. Parker*	15-2548	29.95	26.95
☐ Nursing Theories in Practice *Edited by Marilyn E. Parker*	15-2350	28.95	25.95
☐ Culture Care Diversity & Universality: A Theory of Nursing *Edited by Madeleine M. Leininger*	15-2402	38.95	34.95
☐ On Nursing: A Literary Celebration *By Margretta Styles & Patricia Moccia*	14-2512	29.95	26.95
☐ Transforming RN Education: Dialogue & Debate *Edited by Nancy L. Diekelmann & Marsha L. Rather*	14-2511	39.95	35.95

PHOTOCOPY THIS FORM TO ORDER BY MAIL OR FAX

Photocopy this coupon and send with 1) a check payable to NLN, 2) credit card information, or 3) a purchase order number to: **NLN Publications Order Unit, 350 Hudson Street, New York, NY 10014 (FAX: 212-989-3710).**

Shipping & Handling Schedule

Order Amount	Charges
Up to $24.99	$3.75
25.00-49.99	5.25
50.00-74.99	6.50
75.00-99.99	7.75
100.00 and up	10.00

Subtotal: $ _____

Shipping & Handling (see chart): _____

Total: $ _____

☐ Check enclosed ☐ P.O. # _____ NLN Member # (if appl.): _____

Charge the above total to ☐ Visa ☐ MasterCard ☐ American Express

Acct. #: _____ Exp. Date: _____

Authorized Signature: _____

Name _____ Title _____

Institution _____

Address _____

City, State, Zip _____

Daytime Telephone ( ) _____ Ext. _____